A Major Contribution to the Literature of Parenthood

"In this book, Dr. Elizabeth Whelan has nicely combined a scholarly and personal touch on a subject which is going to become increasingly important as science brings us closer and closer to the day when sex predetermination technology will be a reality."

> —Dr. Charles F. Westoff, Director,
> Office of Population Research,
> Princeton University

". . . demystifies the reproductive process with understandable and accurate information . . . in areas previously left to emotionalism and chance. I would greatly recommend *Boy or Girl?* to all prospective parents."

> —Geraldine Oliva, M.D.,
> Medical Director, Planned Parenthood,
> San Francisco-Alameda

Boy or Girl?

REVISED EDITION

Elizabeth Whelan, Sc.D.

POCKET BOOKS

New York   London   Toronto   Sydney   Tokyo   Singapore

Photographs on pages 87 and 119 appeared in "Sex Control Again" by L. J.
Cole and Ivar Johansson in the *Journal of Heredity*, Volume 24, 1933,
pages 264, and 271.

Revised Edition

POCKET BOOKS, a division of Simon & Schuster Inc.
1230 Avenue of the Americas, New York, NY 10020

ISBN: 978-1-4391-9436-2

First Pocket Books printing January 1986

15   14   13   12   11   10   9

POCKET and colophon are registered trademarks of
Simon & Schuster Inc.

Printed in the U.S.A.

Acknowledgments

I am indebted to a number of people who offered their time and contributed significantly to the research and writing of this book.

Particularly I must express my appreciation to Dr. Rodrigo Guerrero V. of the Universidad del Valle, Division of Health, in Cali, Colombia, who read each draft of this manuscript and offered invaluable comments.

I would also like to thank specifically June Miller for her invaluable research services; Dr. Ronald J. Ericsson, President of Gametrics Limited; Dr. Nancy Williamson of Brown University; Dr. C. G. Vosa of Oxford University; Dr. Peter Barlow of Guy's Hospital Medical School; Sir Alan Parkes of the Galton Foundation; Dr. Don W. Fawcett, Harvard Medical School; and my editors, Stefanie Woodbridge and Mary Heathcote.

I also appreciate the courteous and efficient assistance of the staffs of the New York Academy of Medicine and the New York Public Library.

Contents

Boy or Girl?

Introduction

The Allure of Human Sex Selection

(PAMPHLET CIRCULATED DURING THE EARLY
PART OF THIS CENTURY)

April 1904

Gentlemen:

If you have no son to perpetuate your name, inherit your estates and fortune, why not consult with Mrs. F. M. Foie, a world wide experienced Trained Nurse: she is middle aged, has two handsome sons (gentlemen now). It does not take her twenty minutes to convince her listener of the surety of having his hopes realized . . . and as it (sex pre-determination) rests entirely with him, she objects to consulting with any mother.

Prior to the birth of Mr. Grover Cleveland's third daughter (whom he named after me, Marion, during his last presidency at the White House) I assured Mr. Grover Cleveland that the expected new arrival would be

11

a girl and to his annoyance and great vexation, it was; but since he graciously and so willingly accepted my wonderful never failing experience, two sons have since been born to his great delight and he has ceased further reproach to his amiable wife.

A gardener does not plant an onion and expect a potato to grow from it. I would stake my life if the heir did not appear after my instructions were fully acted upon.

> Respectfully,
> Mrs. F. Marion Foie
> 1810 Amsterdam Avenue
> New York, New York

Mrs. Foie thought she had the answer to an age-old question: how to choose the sex of a child.

I do not know exactly what her answer was, nor do I know how she arrived at it. But I do know that, whatever it was, it was just one of hundreds, maybe thousands, of sex selection methods which have been offered since the beginning of time.

There has always been something intriguing—tantalizing—about the possibility of choosing an unborn baby's sex. But until recently our knowledge in this area was very limited, primarily because the whole topic of human reproduction was surrounded by a cloud of mystery, but also because it is easy to jump to false conclusions when you are dealing with a naturally given set of fifty-fifty odds.

Mrs. Foie, for instance, can point to her own family life and to a few case histories she is familiar with and conclude that she has the ultimate answer. She chooses to ignore the obvious—the fact that any method, no matter how silly or farfetched, will be "successful" about half the time. Similarly, more recent authors in the sex selection field have used informal surveys to "prove" that their advice is effective. Some have actually invited their readers to write in and report on their experiences with the method and the sex of the resulting child. This may be attractive from a human-interest point of view, but, since it is a hopelessly biased sample, it says nothing about the effectiveness of the method. It is a case of "science by vote." Only those who "succeed" are likely to respond.

The only way to determine whether a sex selection method works is, first, to enlist the cooperation of a large number of couples who state a sex preference, and, second, to note the sex outcomes of the pregnancies among couples who have meticulously followed the recommendations. It is critically important that the sex of *all* babies be reported—not just those of parents who volunteer the information in a questionnaire or a thank-you note. Then, if the percentage of boys and girls in this large group deviates significantly from the naturally given 50 percent mark, you have some evidence. This is the *only* type of evidence that is convincing. And this is exactly the type of evidence that *Boy or Girl?* offers.

Expanding interest in sex selection during the past few years has prompted me to update my original book on the topic because I feel that prospective parents deserve to have the very latest information available. They need to know, too, that evidence from ongoing research continues to accumulate in support of the techniques I have recommended, although limitations to those techniques still remain.

Unlike recent sex selection "recipes" that were

based on studies of artificial insemination, *Boy or Girl?* presents information derived from the experiences of hundreds of couples who conceived naturally through sexual intercourse, as most couples do. Additionally, this book offers the only sex selection recommendations that have been repeatedly verified through standard research protocols.

And unlike my predecessors, I will not *guarantee* that you will have a child of the sex of your choice, nor will I even say, as others have, that the method I'll describe is 80 to 90 percent effective. The best I can offer you is a 36 percent greater chance of having a boy or a more modest 16 percent greater chance of having a girl. In other words, if you desire a son, you can increase the odds from fifty-fifty to a maximum of about 68 percent. (The "son" techniques will produce 18 percent more boys, 18 percent fewer girls, for a total of 36 percent greater chance of a boy.) Similarly, the fifty-fifty odds for a girl are raised to 58 percent (8 percent more girls, 8 percent fewer boys).

These figures aren't earth-shaking, but they *are* realistic. With all the smugness befitting a master chef, Mother Nature is still reluctant to divulge all her secrets—regardless of the claims of a few other scientists.

But while the headway made to date is conservative, the light grows slowly brighter. The conclusions presented here remain essentially unchanged since the original publication of this book in 1977, but now there are also ways to up the odds if you are willing to go beyond the bedroom and are able to afford the extra dollars involved. Advances in sperm separation and pharmaceutical products suggest ever-increasing chances for success in years to come. They are certainly important enough to include in the forthcoming chapters, although my major focus continues to be toward helping couples to achieve "success" all by themselves.

As it happens, the most critical portion of this sex selection recommendation contradicts another theory that has become quite well known over the past fifteen years or so. In books and in the popular media, Dr. Landrum B. Shettles and medical writer David Rorvik have eagerly asserted that they have "the one sex selection method that works."

As I will explain in detail in the pages that follow, there is no reason to believe that the so-called Shettles method works. Indeed, by following that sex selection recipe you will actually *reduce* your chances of having a child of the sex of your choice; and if you are seeking a son, you may be inviting medical problems by timing intercourse in a part of the menstrual cycle that is the least favorable for a successful pregnancy—that is, immediately after ovulation. Studies since 1977 dismiss the "Shettles theory" *as it pertains to sexual intercourse*.

My interest in the topic of human sex selection dates back to the late 1960s, when I began doctoral studies at the Harvard School of Public Health. There I met Dr. Rodrigo Guerrero V., a physician who was studying toward a Doctor of Science degree. Dr. Guerrero was analyzing statistics on the sex of babies conceived during various portions of the menstrual cycle, and he began to see some striking patterns that could be useful to couples in planning their families. His subsequent investigations in other parts of the world confirmed that these patterns were real ones, not the kind that could occur by chance. Dr. Guerrero's findings on the timing of intercourse and the sex of offspring were consistent with both animal studies and the relatively few previous studies of couples conceiving naturally. In recent years, his results, based on the largest study of its kind, have been published in the *New England Journal of Medicine, International Journal of Fertility, Studies in Family Planning,* and elsewhere.

It has been known for some years that there is a relationship between sex outcome and the time of insemination within the menstrual cycle. Guerrero's studies showed for the first time that that relationship is very different for couples who conceive naturally and for those who conceive through artificial insemination. I will discuss the reasons why recommendations based on artificial insemination, as the Shettles method is, are not appropriate for attempts to choose the sex of a child conceived in sexual intercourse.

This distinct and very important difference has been the cause of what is an apparent contradiction between the Guerrero and Shettles theories. The point is not so much that the Shettles method is "wrong," but rather that it is "right" *only* for couples who are contemplating artificial methods.

During my own graduate training, I carefully followed the development of research on the subject of sex selection, publishing an extensive review paper on the subject ("Human Sex Ratio as a Function of the Timing of Insemination Within the Menstrual Cycle") in the journal *Social Biology.* But it was after the publication of my book *A Baby? . . . Maybe* that my interest in the area of human sex selection intensified. In that book I explored the quandary many couples today experience about whether or not to have children and how many, if any, to have, offering some specific advice on how to make a comfortable decision about this highly emotional subject.

Soon after publication of the book, I was deluged with requests from couples who needed additional, personal help in making this fateful decision. Very often their questions center on how they might influence the odds of having a child of a given sex. As a result of all these requests I established what I believe was the first preparenthood counseling service, A Baby?. . . Maybe Services, and included among the services sex selection counseling.

No sooner had the service opened its doors than I began to receive more calls, often from scientific and medical colleagues who asked quite bluntly, "Have we figured out the sex determination puzzle yet?" And regularly I received letters, complete with self-addressed stamped return envelopes, from couples who hoped for a son or daughter. Some of these queries were quite casual ("We were just wondering what the latest research in this area was . . ."), but more of them sounded almost panicked ("*Please* let us know by return mail. . . . We want a [son] [daughter] as soon as possible . . ."). When I would mention at a social gathering that I was coordinating A Baby? . . . Maybe Services, I learned not to be at all surprised if an eager couple asked me to summarize Dr. Guerrero's and others' findings right then and there on the back of a cocktail napkin.

After handling a few hundred requests and receiving reports from colleagues who noted first-hand that the Shettles method led to considerable disappointment among patients, I decided that it would be clearer and more convenient for everyone if I set forth in a book the most recent knowledge about human sex selection. Accordingly, I went to South America to work with Dr. Guerrero, the researcher who is now leading the investigation into natural sex selection methods. And I reviewed all the literature on the subject. This book summarizes both historical and current findings in the area of sex selection. It does so in part because perspective is important.

In looking closely at the "how to" of choosing the sex of your child, you should not lose sight of history and of the whole philosophy that lies behind many earlier attempts to select the sex of children. Consider Mrs. Foie's announcement again. In it you can identify three factors that are common to all such historical offers of advice.

First, you'll notice that she promises a son. Indeed, nearly all the "formulas" that have appeared over the years assume that the parents want a male child and that the world would be better off if, as Julian Huxley told the *New York Herald* in 1922, "we [could achieve] the sensational [goal] of relieving the world of its surplus of women." Some commentators explained that it would benefit women if there were more men. For instance, in 1935 Bernarr McFadden and Charles A. Clinton insisted in their *Practical Birth Control and Sex Predetermination* that a preponderance of men was desirable because "naturally there would be fewer sex-starved old maids."

William Roscoe Tucker had the same idea a decade earlier. In his *Do You Wish to Choose the Sex of Children?* he deplored the excess of females because it "entails lack of reverence for womanhood and a consequent lowering of standards of morality." Tucker thought an excess of men could have prevented the Dark Ages, because there would have been enough strength to drive back the attacking plunderers. He recommended, "For the greatest happiness and prosperity there should be more males than females, since a greater number of males are lost through diseases, accidents and wars, and a greater number of males are needed to man the industries of the world."

Second, Mrs. Foie is both enthusiastic and confident, enough so to put her life on the line. Others who "researched" the subject were sure enough of their results to deposit their discoveries in a bank so that they could claim priority. And in one case a would-be sex determinationist took out a copyright on his formula.

Third, Mrs. Foie and others like her are secure in the knowledge that they have a highly desired product to sell. Consider the plight of a middle-aged aristocratic gentleman, a father of six daughters, who in 1904 was discreetly handed Mrs. Foie's literature. He was desperate. He wanted a son and heir. What did he have to lose by trying her advice? He thus entered Mrs. Foie's chambers, and she began her "consultation," knowing well that, unlike other games of chance, hers had a 50 percent probability of winning, no matter what she advised.

Unlike Mrs. Foie, I cannot claim to have all the answers. I cannot stake my life by offering you a guarantee that you won't have a child of the "other sex," no matter what you do. Rather, I admit at the outset that, although we know a great deal about human reproductive physiology and sex determination, we obviously don't know everything.

The quest for the key to human sex selection is different from the search for answers to many other scientific questions. A solution to this riddle has not appeared dramatically—at least not yet. We're not dealing here with a situation in which a white-coated scientist shouts "Eureka!" and triumphantly emerges from his laboratory with the ultimate formula for predicting a boy child or a girl child. Instead, we've gradually accumulated our knowledge about the factors that determine a child's sex, slowly building toward a complete understanding of human reproduction. Ultimately, science may have all the answers. But right now I can bring you only an update on scientific awareness in the area of human sex selection and give you some specifics on how you can apply this knowledge to increase the odds on having a child of the sex of your choice.

I repeat: The most critical portion of this "update" is the revelation that *the "boy and girl recipes" of the late 1960s and early 1970s have now been outdated by new scientific information which contradicts their major assumptions* about the timing of sexual intercourse within the menstrual cycle in order to influence a baby's sex.

I'll begin by looking at some of the underlying reasons why some couples desperately long for a boy or a girl. We are dealing with a very emotional subject. In an age that stresses family planning, it is easy to forget that the desire to have a child is the result of a constellation of psychological needs. Similarly, the feelings about wanting a son or wanting a daughter are also very subtle and complex, perhaps not altogether rational. To get at some of the reasons behind sex preferences, I'm going to introduce you to some of the couples I've talked with in sessions conducted through A Baby? . . . Maybe Services. The comments of the couples quoted have been edited and modified so that they include the most typical attitudes and responses.

I'll then examine the lengths to which some of our predecessors went in their attempts to piece together the sex selection puzzle and after that turn to some of the detailed facts about human reproductive biology, so that you can better understand the advice and thus achieve the desired pregnancy as quickly as possible and with a minimal risk of problems.

But I am also going to introduce some notes of caution: the process of human reproduction cannot be taken for granted. Just as you should not set yourself up for disappointment later by assuming that pregnancy will occur the very month you plan it (this may be particularly true for those who have been using an oral contraceptive, because the natural menstrual pattern usually takes a few months to reassert itself), so *you should be prepared for the possibility that no matter how carefully you apply the current knowledge, you may have a baby of "the other sex."* Right now we have methods that will sway the odds up to 68 percent in your favor. But that still leaves quite a margin for error, and certainly you'll want to be sure that you are willing, indeed eager, to accept the child born to you, whether boy or girl.

One final call for caution. I have given serious consideration to the responsibilities involved in this type of medical research and the implications of truly effective and widespread use of sex determination. I do not overlook the obvious fact that for many couples, and possibly for the world as a whole, sex control may prove to be a mixed blessing. The introduction of a new freedom to choose inevitably brings with it a new burden of decision. Many couples are already faced with deciding whether or not to have children and, if any, how many to have. When the choice of sex distribution in the planned family is added, decision-making will become even more complex, perhaps in some cases bringing a new pressure to the marriage relationship.

Responsible and successful family planning requires

maturity and emotional stability and a general awareness of the implications of one's actions for others.
The delicate natural balance in the sex ratio at birth
may be upset by just one generation that does not
take into account the potential side effects of irrespon-
sible application of new technologies. Human sex control is not an option to be taken lightly. I cannot forget
one worried set of parents who wrote me when they
learned of the work in this area, wondering if "sex
determination is too serious a subject to be left to the
stupidity of man."

I also wonder about that question. My general philosophy here, then, is to proceed in the scientific quest
while at the same time maintaining a healthy respect
for the wisdom of nature's balance.

Elizabeth M. Whelan
New York City

1

So You Want a (Daughter) (Son)

Perhaps you are in the category of those who are planning a first child and think it would be "nice" to have a son (daughter) first. Maybe you want only one child and it is important to you that it be of one particular sex. Possibly you already have one child and are longing for one of the other sex because you know you are going to stop at two. Or perhaps you've had two or more already and are still seeking what you consider the ideal family's sex balance.

There may be medical reasons as well. Researchers have reported nearly 250 different sex-linked genetic disorders. While most are exceedingly rare, two that are probably familiar to most readers are hemophilia and Duchenne's muscular dystrophy, a progressive muscle weakness whose victims require a wheelchair by early adolescence. The genes for both diseases are

23

carried by the female, but affect only male offspring. If parents in such cases are able to produce only daughters, they will avoid the high risk of bearing a child with an incurable disorder. (Approximately 50 percent of all boy babies will be affected by any sex-linked gene carried by the mother.)

If you are interested in what you can do to influence a future baby's sex, your motivations, your circumstances, and the intensity of your desire to have a son or to have a daughter are unique and highly personal. Here I will try to build a framework for analyzing why couples want a child of a particular sex and what that implies in terms of family goals and different attitudes toward the two sexes. But first we should acknowledge that there is another category of would-be family planners, and if you are in this category you may not know about it yet. In today's age of modern contraception and focus on the mechanisms for controlling human fertility, we often forget that some 10 to 20 percent of American couples have difficulty achieving *any* pregnancy, at least for a while. The author is familiar with the couple who seeks advice on sex predetermination, explaining that it is important to them to "start out with a son." After a year or more of trying, they begin to see things quite differently. Or as one woman who discovered she had fertility problems put it, "At this point I don't care if it is a he-she!"

Sons and Daughters

It will come as no surprise to you to learn that, with a few notable exceptions,* throughout history the pref-

---

*For instance, Margaret Mead writes of the Mundugumor, a preliterate cannibalistic people in New Guinea. The Mun-

erence for male children has been significantly stronger than for female children. In many cultures a girl was—and still is—seen as a liability, a burden (especially when it came to finding a husband), possibly even a form of punishment for her parents. The birth of a son, on the other hand, was and still is often seen as an ultimate honor, a reward. Stories that follow show a historical preference for male children and negative attitudes at having only daughters. Dismay over an all-boy family was a rarity.

A few proverbs and traditional sayings will give a flavor of the overwhelming preference for sons. A German adage states, quite colorfully, that "a house full of daughters is like a cellar full of sour beer"; a Japanese proverb laments that "having three daughters is a sure way to stay poor." The Jewish Scriptures tell us that "The Lord blessed Abraham with all—with not having a daughter," and that "He who has not a son is called childless." A Chinese proverb warns that "eighteen goddess-like daughters are not equal to one son with a hump." "May you have a hundred sons" goes the Moslem wedding wish. Girls have been seen as dependents the parents had to marry off. "Daughters are easy to rear but difficult to marry," says a German proverb. "When a good offer comes for a daughter," a Spanish adage advises, "don't wait till her father returns from the market." Anonymous sages counseled, "Marry your son when you will, your daughter when you can," and remarked that "daughters and dead fish are no keeping wares."

But still daughters were born, at about the same rate

dugumor women detest childbearing and child rearing, and the men detest their wives for being pregnant. The men generally resent the birth of a son because the child represents a source of competition.

as sons. So other proverbs were in order. In most cultures there is at least one comforting saying for the new parents of a daughter, along the lines of "That's okay; better luck next time." "A woman of good family always bears a girl as her first child" is the Italian version; "To the lucky man a daughter is first born" is the Spanish one. "It is a good omen when the first baby is a daughter" is the Jewish form of clandestine sympathy.

Why has there traditionally been such a strong desire to have sons?

In earlier centuries there were some good practical reasons to have as many boys as possible. In hunting and gathering societies the birth of a son meant that there was another potential hunter, whereas the birth of a girl merely increased the number of mouths to feed. In circumstances where population growth was outstripping food supply, these societies often turned to the most efficient means of keeping the population of girls in check: female infanticide. Generally the girl babies were not killed directly, but were left to die unattended in the wilderness. In these early cultures life was also extremely hazardous. From adolescence on, men spent much of their time fighting either animals in the hunt or tribes encroaching on their territory. Physical strength and stamina were considered a must for survival, and this spelled a desire for male children.

Second, male children were in the direct line for inheritance of the family land. Indeed, extra sons, who were the "spare parts" in the line of succession, were thought to be necessary because of the high rates of infant and early-childhood death. In many developing countries today—India, for example—this view still lingers. The inheritance factor, as strong for the aristocrat as for the impoverished farmer, here again spawned traditions which have survived to the present day. In Iran, for instance, only a male can succeed as Shah, a practice that could conceivably affect the entire future of a dynasty.

Historically, the most famous example of the strength of a couple's desire to have a son as an heir is that of Anne Boleyn and Henry VIII. Henry annulled his marriage to aging Catherine of Aragon because of his craving for a legitimate male heir to the throne. Anne became pregnant immediately upon their marriage, only to disappoint the anxious king by presenting him with a daughter, Elizabeth. In 1536 Anne did become pregnant with a male child, but it was born dead. Henry then demonstrated his dissatisfaction with his wife by having her beheaded. It was Anne's misfortune that in the sixteenth century the medical books did not explain that it is the male, not the female, whose reproductive cell determines the sex of the child. Even though that fact has been established today, some husbands without sons act much like Henry VIII, presumably not beheading their wives, but rather chiding or even divorcing them for not producing the desired male child.

In the less developed countries of our modern world, sons usually offer the only form of social security for their elderly parents. The economic advantages traditionally offered by a male child have of course been enhanced by the prevailing view that males are the superior of the two sexes. This, along with the desire to have a continuing line of inheritance of family name and property, supports the idea that the world would be better off in every way with a surplus of males.

Evidently, Mother Nature does not concur. Statistics tell us that 120 males are conceived for every 100 females. But a greater number of male pregnancies end in miscarriage, so that only 105 males are actually *born* for every 100 females. After birth, it seems that boys are slightly more susceptible to childhood diseases and other rigors of growing up, so that by reproductive age the numbers are approximately equal. Since the survival rate is so much better for females, one cannot help but wonder which is actually the superior sex.

Why Would a Couple Today Want to Choose the Sex of Their Child?

In the past one could point to some practical—in some cases life-preserving—factors that led prospective parents to wish for boys. But today we do not, at least to the same extent, have these pressures. Women as well as men can and do inherit property. Children of both sexes have nearly equal opportunity in most professions. We are more and more breaking down traditional sex roles, moving toward "unisex" attitudes. Why should contemporary people *care* what the sex of their child is? Could it be true that parents do still have a separate set of attitudes toward and goals for daughters and sons?

This is not a very popular topic to discuss in our age of attempted liberation from sexism, but the fact is that, by definition, a preference for a child of a specific sex does involve some type of sexism, positive or negative. The single exception is the obvious wish to avoid transmitting a known sex-linked genetic disorder to one's offspring. I cannot offer any final judgment about which are "good" and which are "bad" reason to have daughters or to have sons, any more than I can dictate what your personal good or bad reasons to have a baby may be.

In trying to research the whys of sex preference, I turned to dozens of psychology books but could find nothing there. It appeared that scholars had never looked closely at this question. So instead I asked a number of couples the deceptively simple questions, "Why do you want a son?" "Why do you want a daughter?" And I came up with some motivations which you may feel are highly—and in many cases probably rightly—vulnerable to bitter criticism. Frequently they represent gray-haired stereotypes and some strangely distorted concepts about life in general and children in particular. But even in the modern world of the 1980s, these reasons *are* expressed, and couples who are considering choosing the sex of their child may need to deal with them.

JUDY AND DAVID

Judy and David had visions of perfectly planned parenthood. And so far their planning had been successful. Part one of their family plan was to have their first child on or about their fifth anniversary, and they were right on target. Judy left her job as an elementary-school teacher two months before her son, Jamie, was born. Neither Judy nor David had given much thought to the sex of their first child. But that's where part two of their plan comes in. Both of them want their second child to be a daughter, so that they will have what they consider an all-American, well-balanced family.

"We're eager to have our daughter right away," Judy explained as she held her two-year-old son in her lap. "I plan to go back to my teaching job just as soon as

they are both old enough for day care. So I don't want
to spend too much time between births." She spoke
enthusiastically and confidently. There was no doubt in
her mind that the second child would be a girl—all she
wanted from us was the specifics of the "how to."

Judy's blue eyes sparkled as she talked about why
she wanted a daughter. "We'd feel more complete if we
had one of each," she explained slowly, looking over at
David for reinforcement. He simply nodded. "Both of
us are active in Zero Population Growth activities—
I'm head of the education committee and David han-
dles membership. We wouldn't dream of having more
than two. We're all for parenthood—but two's the limit.
And we're so enthusiastic about children that we
wouldn't want to miss the experience of having both a
son and a daughter. Jamie is great. I can't imagine life
without him." She paused for a moment, took a deep
breath, and grinned broadly. "But I really want a
daughter! It would be different! We'd feel deprived if
we didn't have the opportunity to raise a little girl, too.
We want to experience everything! Right, David?"

David nodded again and Judy went on. "You know
all those ads of the 'perfect American Family' always
show a mother and father with a boy and a girl at their
sides. I like that. I think a balanced family is good for
both the parents and the two children. For David and
me it will give us the chance to identify with the child
of our sex, to do all the things we used to do in our own
childhood. We'll get to know what's going on in the Boy
Scout camps *and* we'll eat our share of Girl Scout
cookies!"

David sat forward in his chair. He was considerably
more restrained on the topic than his wife, but he did
have something to add. "I agree," he finally said, "that
it would be exciting to have a daughter. But frankly

don't care all that much what our second child is—as long as he or she is as healthy and bright as Jamie." He looked over at his son and smiled. "But I see Judy's point—I mean, about having the full experience of parenthood. I often wonder whether, if our first child had been a daughter, I wouldn't be the one who was pushing to come over here and talk about sex predetermination.

"But on the other hand, I do see some practical reasons for having a girl next." He laughed and again looked over at his wife and child. "People always told me that a girl was easier to raise. And in the last few months I have begun to see what they mean. I'm a stockbroker and keep strict nine-to-five hours, so it's Judy who's home all day—but I can see that even at this tender age Jamie's full of vitality and mischief." Jamie seemed to react to this, throwing his well-worn stuffed animal in the direction of his father. "I think one son is great, but I am ready for a daughter. She'll be calmer, and a good change of pace from Jamie. I think the real differences there will show up in those terrible teen years. Boys get wild—I remember what it was like, let me tell you."

Judy threw back her head and laughed. "I second that. I've watched Jamie in the park where there are little girls his age. And there is a difference in behavior. I've got to keep after Jamie every minute. Yes, I'll be ready for a change too."

MIMI AND BRIAN

Brian and Mimi had strong ideas about the sex of the one child they planned to have. The problem was that their ideas did not mesh. He wanted a son. She wanted a daughter.

Brian refused to talk about his feelings, but Mimi

was eager to explain. "When we were married two years ago, we agreed that we'd wait awhile, but we basically agreed that we'd have at least one. It's only recently that we really began to hash the subject out, and now we've got a problem. You see, the way I look at it is that it's in everyone's best interest that we have just one. We both teach at the university and enjoy our professional lives. On that we agree. But I really want a daughter—and he's all hung up on some machismo trip." She shook her head angrily. "He can't explain why he wants a son. He just says 'because.' But I have my reasons for a daughter."

She sat back in the chair and folded her arms. "I'll admit that the women's movement has a lot to do with my feelings. I think a woman's time has finally come. Today it is truly exciting to be a female—and I think things will be even better when my daughter is grown. My goodness! I'm talking about her as if she existed." She laughed at herself and went on. "I would delight in sharing in the life of a daughter—helping her through the rough spots of adolescence, seeing her triumph over all the sexist obstacles that I had to fight. I guess what I'm saying is that I could identify more with a girl; we'd have so much more of life to share.

"And there's another thing too. A girl is more permanent." Mimi considered this statement for a moment and went on. "I can imagine a son taking off on his own for months at a time without even dropping us a line. I think a daughter keeps in touch with you more. I know that's the way it is in our family. My brother usually forgets my parents' birthdays. He's off in his own world. But I talk to my parents a few times a week, even though they live almost a thousand miles away.

"I've told Brian my feelings. But he's impossible on

the subject. We've even considered a compromise—
two children, one of each. But that doesn't satisfy him
either! He insists the son has to be born first! And I say
'no way.' I really don't know how we are going to work
this out."

ELLEN AND STEVE

Ellen and Steve were very subdued when they spoke
of their interest in sex selection. Ellen, a reserved
woman, described herself as a "stay-at-home house-
wife and mother." Steve explained that he owned and
ran a service station and automobile repair shop in a
small town. "We were married pretty late," Steve began. He seemed a bit uncomfortable talking about the
subject. "We were in our late twenties, and, well, really
turned on about the idea of having kids right away. Our
baby, Jackie, arrived a year later—and we couldn't have
been happier. Then . . ."

Ellen interrupted cautiously. "Dear, maybe I should
explain that part. We didn't want to waste any time
having our second, because I was almost thirty—and
then it didn't happen. I mean I didn't get pregnant."
She shut her eyes and shook her head slowly. "Finally,
after four years of trying, I did conceive—and two
months ago we were blessed with another daughter.
And I do mean blessed!" Ellen spoke a bit defensively.
"Our problem is that now I am thirty-five, and we don't
have a son yet." She turned to Steve, her eyes asking
him to pick up the conversation.

"I think the guys at the shop would stop teasing me
if we had a son." He laughed a bit, and then suddenly
became serious. "The day our second daughter was
born, every one of them had a wisecrack: 'Hey, what's
going on? Don't you believe in boys in your family?'

'Can't quite muster up enough strength, hey, fellah?' "
Steve frowned. "It's almost as if something were wrong
with me for not having a son. And I'll admit it—I would
feel better, well, as a man, if we did have one. I'd love to
go into the garage one day with cigars that said 'It's a
boy!' That'd show 'em I could do it!" He smiled briefly
and then turned serious again. "Don't get me wrong. I
love my daughters, and I'm mighty proud of them. But
oh, God, I wish we had a son!" Steve was speaking
slowly and fervently now. "I'd also love to call my own
father someday and say, 'Guess what, Dad, I've got a
son of my own.' " Ellen and Steve smiled sadly at each
other. "It's hard to describe," Steve went on, "but I
just feel it would round out my life to have a boy of my
own. I'd be complete. Do you understand that?"

"I do," Ellen volunteered in a soft voice, looking at
her husband with sympathy. "I can't help but see a bit
of myself in my two daughters. They're extensions of
me—they make me feel more complete as a person—as
a woman. I'm sure Steve would feel the same way
about his son—if we had one." Her voice trailed off,
and she began to stare at the floor.

Steve returned to the conversation. "Okay. There's
something else. I know it's trite—but a boy does carry
on the name. If it's just the two girls, that will be the end
of my family. I'd be the last link in the chain. And that
makes me feel pretty bad. Family has always been
important to me—to all of us—and a boy offers a
chance for that." He thought a moment. "I think the
point is that boys are more permanent. Girls join someone else's family. A son has got your name, and he is
always your son. Your daughter changes her name and
goes from being your daughter to being someone else's
wife!"

Ellen wasn't paying attention to what Steve was saying. She was deep in her own thoughts, and obviously on the verge of tears. Her face reflected pain as she said, "I had an abortion the year before we were married. Steve and I weren't ready for children yet. I keep thinking it might have been a boy . . ."

EMILY AND BILL

Emily and Bill were married for nine years before they began to resolve the question of whether or not to have children. "We are both committed to our jobs," Emily explained. She spoke in a formal, businesslike tone. "We just didn't know whether it was financially feasible to handle both parenthood and careers. We didn't know whether it would be fair to a child. I'm an account executive with a public relations group here in the city, and I travel very frequently." She shook her head as if to emphasize the point.

"So we went over the pros and cons, and we finally decided yes," Bill added. "We know it's going to be tough. We're both going to keep our jobs, if we can swing it. Emily has agreed to cut her traveling back, and thank goodness my job—I'm a dentist—gives me some flexibility. I'm hardly ever out of town." He smiled and clasped Emily's hand. "I just hope we haven't waited too long. Emily's been using the Pill for nine years and . . ."

"The point is," Emily said, making it clear she wanted to keep the meeting on target, "that we want just one child—and we both feel it should be a boy. We've talked a lot about it." She shifted around in her chair and then, for the first time, laughed and looked more relaxed. "My goodness! It seems that the baby question is about all we've talked about for the last five years! But when we finally decided to go ahead, some-how we both knew that a son was our choice. And I'll tell you why." She took a deep breath and spoke in a way which left no doubt that this topic had been given a great deal of thought. "A boy is more achievement-oriented," she said. "We're not exactly what you'd call sexist people, but we want our only child to be a son, because Bill and I ourselves are hard workers, always striving for success, and we want our child to follow in our footsteps."

"Yeah," Bill agreed. "I know this is the age of women's liberaton, but somehow we both feel more comfortable about transferring our values to a son. We would take great pleasure in watching our child take up a career in law, medicine, business, maybe he'll even want to be a dentist—or whatever. You know, a girl could decide she wanted to quit after high school and get married and have children. We'll have a better chance for our views of success with a son."

"And there's another thing . . ." Emily paused and for a moment spoke directly to Bill. "We haven't really talked about this, but I think it's particularly important for me." She took a few seconds to organize her thoughts and went on. "When we have our baby, it's my life that will change the most. I know Bill will help out. But more of the responsibilities will fall on me. And since I am not willing to give up my job—just the travel—I want to have a child who's easy to raise. You don't have to worry about boys as much. It seems to me that girls would need more of your time. Of course boys are probably more of a hassle, especially early on, but they go out on their own more quickly. That's why I think . . ."

Bill interrupted. "Yes. A good point. I can imagine

being concerned about a daughter even after she's married. Somehow she is always your responsibility. You have to look out for her more."

SANDRA AND PETER

Sandra and Peter were married immediately after high-school graduation, and their first child, a son, was born six months after the wedding. "You get the picture," Peter commented hastily, "but it all worked out for the best. And we had our second boy two years later." He was eager to get to the main topic of conversation. "Let me tell you our problem. We're having real troubles right now making ends meet—the economy and all—and I've been laid off at the plant a few times in the past few years. Everyone who knows us thinks we've had our two kids, and that since we're hardly millionaires, we'll stop. But we want a daughter—we really do. And that's both of us!"

"I'm so happy that Peter feels that way too," Sandra said quietly. "I feel cheated that I don't have a daughter. Frankly, I look enviously at my friends' children, and they tell me, 'Sandy, you're really missing out.' I mean, girls are different." She sighed, "Oh, I guess we were like everyone else. We wanted a boy first, and of course we were thrilled with our first son even though he wasn't exactly . . . uh . . . planned. But during the second pregnancy I hoped and prayed it was a girl. I went shopping for little pink clothes, all kinds of dainty things. I convinced myself I was carrying a girl." She shook her head and then said seriously, "The feelings were so strong that day my second son was born, I felt as if I'd lost a child as well as gained one.

"Girls are different!" she said again. "I would just love to take care of a daughter, to brush her hair, buy her bright ribbons, colorful dresses, Somehow I think she could be more of a companion to me; I could be closer to her; she would confide in me about her personal problems more than I expect my sons will. I really want to have a daughter!"

Peter nodded. "I know it's not stylish to say so, but girls are somehow softer, more sensitive. I think I would like to have a little girl to take care of. She'd look up to me in a much more dependent way than my sons do." He looked a bit sheepish as he added, "I never really thought about this before, but I guess I'd even enjoy giving the bride away once in my lifetime!"

Commonly Expressed Reasons for Wanting a Boy or Wanting a Girl

Wanting a Son	*Wanting a Daughter*
A son is more permanent	A daughter is more permanent
A boy is an easier child to raise	A girl is an easier child to raise
A son will carry on the family name	A girl is someone you can take care of
Boys are more achievement-oriented	It's easier to raise someone of your own sex
I'd feel more like a man	A woman's time has come. It's exciting to have a daughter today

Wanting at Least One of Each Sex

We'd feel more complete as a family
We want to have the experience of both

Is There a "Difference"?

Are there really innate differences in behavior between the sexes? Obviously there is no definitive answer to that question, and different parents offer different opinions.

Plato would evidently have agreed that a girl is an easier child to raise; he wrote that "of all animals, the boy is the most unmanageable . . . of all the wild beasts, the most difficult to manage." Various daffy definitions of the "boy" include "a noise with dirt on it," "a cross section between a god and a goat," "an appetite with a skin pulled over it," and "one who has a wolf in his stomach," all of which would support the view of some couples that boys are more "difficult" children (and certainly hungrier).

Messages on those "congratulations on your new baby" cards found in every stationery department and store long supported the popular assumption (without benefit of facts) that boys are harder to manage, capable of wearing out even the most energetic of parents. As recently as five years ago, the following verses were typical greeting card fare:

> A boy is a mischievous, magical marvel,
> An angel with mud on his face . . .

> A little boy
> Who makes more noise
> And plays more pranks
> Attracts more dirt
> Deserves more spanks . . .

Other verses mention pockets full of turtles, beetles, grasshoppers, pebbles, and snails, and various episodes of immersion in mud puddles. This aspect of childhood is not mentioned much in the cards for a girl baby. She is depicted as a dainty, well-behaved angel:

> So God created little girls
> With laughing eyes and bouncing curls . . .
>
> Sweet as a sugar plum,
> Soft as a dove,
> A bundle from heaven
> To pamper and love.

Evidently some feminist group or other must have set about correcting what millions of parents can attest were whopping misconceptions. For the most part, card writers of the mid-1980s have abandoned the chauvinistic approach in favor of equal opportunity. As many as always still designate "baby girl" or "baby boy" on the front, but in roughly three-quarters of them (in an unofficial survey) the verses are either identical or contain such non-committal lines as:

> A baby girl is
> life's most precious gift.

and

> He's sunshine, he's laughter,
> He's your pride and joy
> And he's extra special,
> He's your little boy.

Adages and cards aside, there is no good reason to assume that a child of one or the other sex will be more difficult. Certainly attitudes and expectations, unique discipline patterns, and other factors may make boys more unruly, but the notion that males are naturally more troublesome and girls naturally more docile and sweet-tempered belongs in the album of old wives' tales and sexist myths.

Sons, Daughters, Motivations

When the motivations of those first five couples interviewed are considered, a few points become clear. First, many, if not most, people *do* have different feelings about sons and daughters. That may not mean that they think one sex is "better" than the other; it's just that they think raising a son is a different experience from raising a daughter. Second, in wanting a child of a particular sex, many men and women have stereotypes in mind: the boy as the achiever, the girl as the dainty dependent princess. Third, many of the motivations for wanting to have a girl (or a boy) baby—like many of the reasons for having children in general—are based on subtle psychological needs.

And sometimes these needs are not so subtle, as in the case of Lola and Tim, who brought me a somewhat different type of problem. They were hoping—almost insisting—that their intended only child would be a girl. After chatting for a few minutes it was apparent that Tim would be content either way, but Lola was adamant.

"I have *four brothers,*" she wailed, "and I've never really gotten along well with any of them for long. Even today I don't like them very much. Growing up with all those little boys was plain awful and apparently they intended it should stay that way." After reflecting a moment, Lola's voice grew quieter and assumed a confidential note. "I'm not quite sure how to say this, but I've had a really massive problem relating to the opposite sex ever since I can remember. Tim is one of the few males I've ever felt really comfortable with. So naturally," she added with a nervous giggle, "I let him catch me as soon as possible! But now . . . the very *thought* of having to be around another little boy again totally terrifies me! I know that's not quite rational, but I just can't shake it, and we do really want a baby. A few of my closer friends have suggested I see a therapist or someone to get rid of my hangup. But that seems like such an unnecessary extravagance when I feel that I'm basically well-adjusted in other respects."

I glanced at Tim who was nodding agreement and he shrugged his shoulders at me. "I have nothing to add except to tell you that what Lola says is true. We have a marvelous relationship, and there's no doubt that she's a happy, relaxed sort of person—except for the baby issue." Their expectant faces were begging for some miraculous solution.

I explained to them that, although I could outline the procedures for increasing their chances at having a girl, the performance of miracles was outside my domain, and I could not even pretend that this would solve their problem. Yet I saw there a very warm, loving young couple, intelligent and concerned, who appeared to be ideal candidates for parenthood. I cannot recall my exact words but my speech to them went something like this:

"To begin with, I have no 100-percent-effective magic formula, no money-back guarantee. Let's suppose that Mother Nature refuses to cooperate and you give birth to a son. What then? Even suppose that as you view this angelic little bundle cooing in his crib you feel your fears slip away and vow that you will always adore him no matter what. How about when he's two years old and, on a particularly bad day, spends twelve straight hours alternately ransacking the house and throwing temper tantrums—how are you going to deal with that? Will you simply react with justifiable anger at his misbehavior, or will you become furious with him and blame it all on the irrefutable fact that he's a *boy*?"

They listened intently as I reminded them that the 1980s have ushered in a quite different culture from the one most of us in the new-parent generation knew as children. The first tentative steps toward male-female "equality" began in the 1960s, flourished in the 1970s, and are now settling into a new and accepted way of life. There are still wrinkles to smooth and hassles to deal with, certainly. But aside from anatomical structure, the differences between Man and Woman are decreasing by the week. For Lola and Tim—especially for Lola—I stressed the important implications of these trends.

I then asked them the same question that I now pose to you: *What exactly is it that you expect from a daughter that could not be fulfilled by a son? Or, if the converse applies, from a son rather than a daughter?*

If you expect a little girl who prances around in a white pinafore, happily giggling but never misbehaving, you might as well spend your money on a Cabbage Patch doll. A real-life daughter of the 1980s and 1990s will likely as not be able to throw as mean a spitball as anyone in the neighborhood, after which she will forget to wash behind her ears, and sit down to prepare for another A on her algebra homework—while her brother will return from his ballet lesson to help prepare dinner for the family and then curl up with a good book of poetry. The old stereotypes are joining the ranks of the horse and buggy.

While adults tend to be relatively slow in accepting

and adjusting to the changing scene, today's children are being born into it. Acknowledging that there will always be some exceptions (as there have always been), modern-day youngsters are as disinclined to adopt the role of "typical" boy or girl as their great-grandparents are to accept the word "unisex."

I am generally reluctant to advise psychological counseling for two major reasons: first, because many people misunderstand and become offended; second, because it sounds too much like a cop-out: "I can't—or won't—be responsible for your problem; let someone else do it." But in this case there were factors that transcended my reluctance. I did suggest to Lola that she might benefit from some form of counseling, simply because her specific problem was more deep-seated than the simple lack of awareness of a changing culture. But I *also* recommended she try babysitting for very short periods of time with some of her friends' young sons in the hope that familiarity might drive away some of her fear.

For most people, however, the key to resolving many of the old perceptions of boy-girl differences lies in a simple willingness to accept the world as it is right now, rather than the way you were probably brought up to expect it should be.

Sue Ann and Mike had mastered this concept very well. Already young parents of a three-year-old daughter, they almost sparkled as they began their story. "We've been talking a lot since Sue Ann first called you," Mike began, "and I think we reached some important conclusions on our own. But since we had the appointment anyway we wanted to sound them out with you."

Sue Ann picked up. "We started exploring in depth

our reasons for wanting a son the next time around. As soon as we got past the obvious all-American-family/one-of-each concept, we realized we had been caught up in issues that no longer exist. When I sort of tentatively brought that up to Mike, he just stared at me for an hour-long minute. I thought I had really offended him in some way. Then he burst out laughing."

"I had been thinking along the very same lines," Mike chimed in, "and I was trying to figure out how to mention it without hurting Sue Ann's feelings." He grinned. "Fortunately, she's always been more outspoken than I."

"Now we can concentrate on more relevant things like whether to move to a larger apartment or redecorate the one we have," Sue Ann continued with a wink. "No hassles about pink or blue booties."

We continued the discussion for quite some time, during which they expressed so much enthusiasm and simple wisdom that by the time they bubbled out I had almost come to feel it was they who had earned the consultation fee.

Expectations

Do you have a better chance for great achievement with a son? Possibly. Then on the other hand, maybe not. But in many people's minds boys do have a greater prospect of "doing things" with their lives. In those earlier greeting cards, boys were almost always portrayed as being active—climbing trees and fences, riding bikes, and generally breezing along on the road to success ("for whatever the challenge, a boy's willing to try," "to conquer the seas, explore the plains," "he's all of your hopes for a bright future").

Of course, while the boys were out conquering the world, the girls were, according to those cards, soft, cuddly, responsive, ("the sweet and precious thing you love, sweet as a sugar plum, soft as a dove," "so innocent and sweet," "sugar sweet with just a dash of spice"), full of fun and laughter ("a girl is all giggles and glamour and grace"), and an object you can dress in bright frilly things ("satin bows and ruffly dresses").

Such conventional notions didn't necessarily jibe with reality—nor did they in our grandparents' era. With the passing years, women have successfully "invaded" almost every profession and trade, albeit many of them are still frustrated with a certain amount of discrimination, however subtle. Complaints are not infrequent that a woman has to work "twice as hard as a man" to achieve the same goals, but the ladies have persisted, nonetheless, and presumably the future will bring true equality. It is the stereotype that is difficult to shake.

Needs

When couples like the ones described earlier tell you that they want a son "to carry on the family name" or "to feel like a man," or that they want a daughter "to take care of" or, in the case of a mother, "to delight in sharing the life of a daughter," they are expressing some basic human need, perhaps in a disguised form.

Do sons make a man feel more masculine, or make him feel that he will live on through his name? It appears that many men do indeed believe that a son will meet such needs, and that many women, aware of how much a son means to their husbands, may themselves take on the fervent desire to have a male child. In some countries the macho idea is more prevalent than in the United States. In Puerto Rico, for example, a man who fathers female children is often teased and called a *chancletero*, which literally means "maker of cheap slippers." Occasionally the birth of a female child is seen as a punishment, and the father's friends may comment, "That is to pay for your sins."

And as for "continuing the name," a son—unlike a daughter, who may marry and leave the family setting—may be viewed as a passport to immortality. But here, too, trends are changing. For years it has not been uncommon for women in business to continue using their maiden names for professional purposes. Traditionally, movie stars, stage actresses, musicians, artists, and writers have retained their names. Today more and more married women are not assuming their husbands' names at all (resulting in an occasional raised eyebrow as spectators are left to contemplate whether the couple is "really married"). Generally the children of such marriages are given a hyphenated surname that combines the last names of both parents. The result may be long-winded at times, but it does solve the family-name problem.

Then, too, even a quarter-century ago, I was acquainted with a couple wherein *he* took *her* name and, as far as I know, everyone (including their two sons) has lived happily ever after.

There are two more needs that may be reflected in a desire to have a son or to have a daughter. A child of the same sex offers a parent the opportunity to relive much of his or her own childhood experience. Psychiatrists call this phenomenon "unfolding," that is, reliving, and to some extent revising, events of earlier life, often resolving conflicts in the process. The parent who wants a child of his or her own sex may, consciously or not, want to relive or revise some specific experiences.

(Mimi was explicit here, wanting a daughter so that she could see her offspring grow up without the prejudices she had faced as a female.) Similarly, part of the desire of a father for a son may be the fact that he can identify closely with and enjoy vicariously the child's experiences.

"I think I would like to have a little girl to take care of," Peter told me. Parents of children of both sexes often describe as one of the joys of parenthood the fact that their children make them feel very special, very needed. But possibly this feeling may be even stronger among men who want daughters. The role of guardian may appeal to a father and play an important role in his desire to have a girl child. A Spanish proverb summarizes it: "He who has daughters is always a shepherd." "A daughter is to her father a treasure of sleeplessness" is another adage. A man's feeling of responsibility for a daughter's welfare may not be a burden but rather a joy. A father may also see a daughter as being more sensitive, more emotionally generous. As Euripides wrote, "To an old father, nothing is more sweet than a daughter; boys are more spirited, but their ways are not so tender." But Euripides wrote that more than 2,000 years ago.

The "Wrong" Sex

With some couples I interviewed, the desire for sex selection was already adamant. Ginny, mother of three sons, flatly told me, "Some people manage to have at least one of each but we give up—the thought of possibly raising *four* boys is just too overwhelming!"

Kay and Don, on the other hand, were the parents of three daughters. "All the girls are on softball teams," Kay told me wistfully. "Don is always there cheering at their games, but underneath he still considers it a creampuff sport, compared to baseball. Two of the girls are also cheerleaders during football season. He never misses one of those games either, but I sometimes catch him watching the rough-and-tumble play on the field with a sad expression on his face, and I know he feels a little like he's been cheated. That's not quite logical, of course. We both realize that the birth of a son doesn't necessarily mean the birth of a star quarterback. But it would have been nice if we could have had a chance to find out."

I am personally acquainted with both families and know that the parents are highly involved with their children, and that they are essentially progressive, equality-minded thinkers. With deep sincerity they frequently mention how very fortunate they feel to have three healthy, bright children. Yet inescapably there is the whiff of a void in their lives.

But while most families manage to adapt to the distribution at hand, some seem to have programmed themselves for disaster.

Brenda and Jerry were delighted with their female first-born. But with the birth of their second daughter four years later, Jerry took no pains to hide his disappointment. He continued to lavish attention on the older girl but would have nothing to do with the second, as though it were somehow her own fault that she had been born the "wrong" sex.

Such cases are worse than sad. Without some type of intervention and redirection, the lives of an entire family can be needlessly shrouded in pain. This is why I shall risk growing tiresome as I repeatedly admonish you to examine your personal motives and attitudes concerning sex selection. If your specific desire is so powerful that you question your ability to cope adequately with disappointment, there are two possible routes.

First, you need to go back and seriously review your reasons for wanting a child—or another child—at all. When the miracle of life is forced to take a back seat to the miracle of life *of a particular sex,* it indicates a confusion of priorities. My intention is not to make you feel guilty about your personal preferences. I wish only to point out that where there exists a really deep-seated, almost uncontrollable longing for a child of a particular sex, and you are unable to reconcile it, no matter how hard you try, you may wish to consider the alternative solution of adoption. It is the only sure way to realize your dreams.

There is a caveat here as well. Many years ago there were more babies waiting to be adopted than there were parents who wanted them. But trends have gradually tipped the balance into a drastically opposite situation. Legalized abortion; increased use of effective, easily available contraception; and the fact that many unwed mothers now choose to keep their babies and "go it alone," if necessary, have greatly reduced the number of babies available for adoption. My sources tell me that, because this scarcity has so prolonged the waiting period, most prospective parents are more than eager to accept a baby of *either* sex. When a specific request is made, most agencies are willing to acknowledge it, but with the understanding that it may take even longer than the usual two years or more for the "right" baby to become available.

I find it particularly interesting that with current surveys indicating an overwhelming preference for male babies—even today, when it would seem the difference should be less marked—this same preference does not generally extend into adoption agency requests. Even in our sophisticated era of technology, the old adage keeps popping into mind about the fellow who complained of no shoes until he met a man with no feet.

A moderate preference for either a boy or a girl is natural, understandable, and acceptable. When desperation creeps on the scene, the picture changes radically. And so I repeat: medical science can help you increase the odds, but *it can offer no guarantees.* And since the chances are still relatively high that you may give birth to the "wrong" sex, both you and your spouse need to consider seriously what kind of reaction is likely to result. If you are certain—that is, as certain as you are able to be in dealing with a hypothetical issue—that neither of you will suffer more than minimal disappointment, here's wishing you all the best.

Even the slightest doubt, however, raises the question of just what it is you are expecting to gain from parenthood. Few couples are able, much less willing, to reply to that one with a truly definitive answer. And that's all right, too, at least most of the time. As I discussed at length in *A Baby? . . . Maybe,* the "right" reasons for some may be totally "wrong" for others. My concern really has little to do with ethical relativity per se, but rather what is right or wrong for you *and your child*. If the decision to have a baby (or another baby) is based on answers like "Yes, if it's a girl" or "We only want a boy," these are bright red flashers warning of decidedly unrealistic expectations. Take some time to think over the following:

• How will I feel if our baby is not the sex we preferred? Will I still be able to offer him/her the same amount of love, attention, and patience? Will my spouse?

• Will I be able to conquer any disappointment adequately so that it is never transmitted to my child?

• In the years ahead will I be able to face the moments of adversity without the temptation to mourn, "If only you'd been the other sex!"

• Am I willing to acknowledge that the most "masculine" male is capable of decorating a cake or sewing on a button as neatly as any female, and that, other things being equal, a female can drive a truck or design a bridge with the same potential success as a male?

Perhaps in earlier years you always felt more comfortable around boys and thus vaguely believe the same attitude will linger into parenthood. (Think about it: Do you still feel uncomfortable around other females? Even if you do, do you honestly think this would affect your attitude toward a daughter?)

Perhaps you've always melted at the sight of little-girl clothes and can't wait to dress up your own youngster. (Take a look around. Unless it's a very special occasion, you won't see many girls, not even infants, in pink ruffles and lace tights.)

Perhaps like many other youngsters, you grew up with a preconceived notion of how your family would be put together. A typical blueprint specified a boy first "to look after his younger sister," who would be born exactly two years later, and so on. Twenty or thirty years ago, that line of thinking might have had a little merit, although not much. Today it really makes no sense at all.

Introspection

There are three vital points to keep in mind as you carefully attempt to analyze your feelings: 1) that you try to be completely honest with yourself about your motivations (after all, no one needs to know your answers but you); 2) that you attempt to place your motivations into reasonable perspective; and 3) that you are prepared for the possibility that you may give birth to a child of the "other" sex. If "failure" is an unacceptable alternative, perhaps you ought not to attempt pregnancy at all.

Since the first edition of *Boy or Girl?* was published, some incredibly sad letters have crossed my desk. Many of them carry the theme of "We thought it wouldn't matter but it does!" Other letters are irate ones from couples who tried the Guerrero "recipe" and it didn't work. Since I never promised otherwise, I do not feel guilt but rather relief that I do not have to be the subject of their wrath on a daily basis. (I can only hope that by directing their anger at me it consequently bypasses the child.)

On the subject of letters I hasten to point out that there are many, many happy ones as well. While I do not profess to be responsible for all of their "successes," perhaps none of them at all, it nevertheless pleases me to think that I might have played some small role in contributing to their joy. That, after all, is the underlying purpose of this book.

Attitudes toward parenthood are emotionally based, and the desire or nondesire for children in general—and for boy or girl children in particular—may stem from deep within the psyche. As the failure to have children can evoke guilt feelings or resentment toward the spouse, so can the failure to have a child of the desired sex, even though those feelings are physiologically unwarranted. Among couples who have two or three children of one sex and long for a child of the other, memories of a past abortion can have tormenting effects. The "what if" thoughts are quite similar to those of now infertile women who had abortions earlier.

While the focus of this book is sex selection, the focus of this chapter has been the motivation behind the desire for sex selection. I cannot conclude this discussion without acknowledging a factor that many researchers in the areas of sex predetermination and sex preference overlook. In some studies couples are given a deck of four cards, two that say "boy," two that say "girl"; the husband and wife are asked to "deal" them in the order they perceive as representing an ideal family. What this research protocol omits is a card that says "child." Not everyone has strong feelings about having a boy first or having a girl first, or even about having a balanced family.

"We Want a (Girl) (Boy)! What Are We Going to Do About It?"

With some understanding of the feelings that can lead a couple to want to choose the sex of their children, we can proceed to the "how to." I will preface the description of the latest knowledge about human sex predetermination with some of the "tried but not necessarily true" methods of the past. These attempts of yesteryear give us some evidence of how strong the motivation for sex control has been. They also offer considerable insight into the complexities of human nature and the intricacies of the male-female relationship.

.

2

Methods That Work— About Half the Time

Try to imagine yourself living several thousand or even a few hundred years ago. You didn't understand how pregnancy occurred or what the human reproductive process was all about. You might have suspected that pregnancy was the result of sexual intercourse, but then again there was some fairly strong evidence that you were wrong. Very young girls and older women had sex, yet they didn't become pregnant. Some women had regular intercourse for twenty or thirty years and never had a baby. Perhaps, as some around you claimed, childbearing, like menstruation, was just another peculiarly female event that men had nothing to do with. Pregnancy "just happened"—and very mysteriously.

On the other hand, if you accepted the more traditional beliefs in this area, perhaps you thought that it was women who had only a very small role in reproduction. Many ancient Egyptians and others felt that the female body was just the place where the male seed, complete unto itself, grew. Thus they felt free to use females captured in war as concubines, because they believed the resulting offspring would have no taint of foreign blood; the woman was merely an "accessory."

It is worth noting, however, that at some point the early Egyptians must have had at least some knowledge of reproduction. James Breasted, the noted Egyptologist, has translated a hymn to the sun-god Aten, written about 1400 B.C. It begins:

Creator of the germ in woman,
Maker of seed in man,
Giving life to the son in the body of his mother . . .

We also know that they were acquainted with bird incubation as early as 3000 B.C. Why so relatively little was written by this highly advanced civilization about anatomy and physiology is something of a puzzle, but we can safely speculate that religious restriction played an important role. Indeed, this is probably the major reason that the human reproductive process remained shrouded in mystery for so long. Only well into the twentieth century did the most basic facts come to light.

Until 1930 it was the prevailing belief that ovulation—the release of the egg from the ovary—occurred during the days of menstrual bleeding. Female dogs experienced bleeding when they were in "heat," that is, on the days mating and conception took place. This information was believed to apply equally to humans.

It was in 1929–30 that two researchers, one Japanese (Dr. Kyusaku Ogino) and the other German (Dr. Herman Knaus), working independently, noted that menstruation and ovulation are two separate events.

Not understanding the basics of reproduction, but being highly motivated by practical necessities or strong emotions to plan your future child's sex, how would you have gone about it in an earlier century? You'd probably have reached the same conclusion the ancients did: "Anything is worth a try." Add to this "try anything" approach the belief that males were superior beings, and you have the basis for the historical means of sex preselection.

Predicting the Unpredictable

Before we focus on some of the traditional means of influencing sex outcome, let's consider the methods the ancients used to predict sex outcome once pregnancy had occurred.

Some of these methods were relatively sophisticated, even though we now know they have no scientific basis. For instance, an Egyptian papyrus, one of our earliest known medical records, advised a urine test for women who suspected they were pregnant: "To see if a women is pregnant or not pregnant, barley and wheat are moistened daily with the woman's urine, like dates or pastry in two bags. If either germinate, so will she give birth. If the wheat germinates, so will it be a boy; if the barley germinates, so will it be a girl; if they do not germinate, so she is not pregnant."

This general idea of the do-it-yourself pregnancy test had found its way into European medical circles by the seventeenth century. The general rule then was, "Make two holes in the ground, in one place some wheat, in the other barley, wet with the woman's urine and cover with earth. If the wheat sprouts first, the woman has a male fetus; if the barley first, a female."

But most pregnancy-predicting techniques of the past were not quite so laboratory-oriented. Generally it was believed that you could just look at the prospective mother, ask her a few questions, and you'd have the answer.

Albertus Magnus, in his widely used medieval medical text *De Secretis Mulierum,* wrote that a woman carrying a boy would have marked changes on the right, or superior, side of her body: her right breast would be larger, with dark, pigmented surface areas around her nipple, and this breast would tend to secrete milk earlier. Her right eye would be brighter, the pupil larger and with more sparkle, and her right nostril would bleed frequently. Since males were believed to be more fully developed than females, they would certainly move in the womb earlier. Aristotle claimed that for boys, "quickening" occurred earlier. Interestingly, this distinction provided the basis for the Roman Catholic Church's early rulings on abortion. Although there has always been universal agreement in the Church that abortion is murder, the exact moment at which the fetus is infused with a rational soul—and thus the definition of "murder"—was not always clear. Up to 1869 almost all of the Church fathers accepted Aristotle's view that the soul developed in various stages, only becoming "rational" or "animated" after some weeks of gestation, specifically forty days after conception for a male fetus, eighty to ninety days for a female. How the prenatal "determination" of sex was arranged is not known.

Not only would women carrying a son notice "right" symptoms, but historical medical records reflect the prevailing belief that these women would be more likely to develop headaches, mistiness before the eyes, a distaste for food, and a "rising stomach," since they were carrying something "foreign" inside them. On the other hand, because of the widely held assumption that male babies generated warmth, a mother soon to deliver a son would glow with health, while a woman carrying a daughter would be pallid and listless. If a woman's expanding abdomen was high, round, and prominent, the child would surely be male; if her profile was egg-shaped and drooping, a daughter was on the way.

An ancient Japanese belief held that the sex of a family's future child could be predicted from the nuchal hair (hair at the nape of the neck) of the child born directly before it. When the hairs converged, the next child would be a girl; when they diverged, a boy. Lest you think that this is ancient hogwash that would not be considered by modern men, I must point out that a report in a 1911 issue of the *Journal of Anatomy* concluded that this method was "85 percent correct" and suggested that further research be done in this area. Indeed, despite the fact that they have no scientific basis, many of the historical sex prediction methods mentioned here are part of our contemporary folklore. Some women still tell their obstetricians that they "just know" it's a boy because they have more morning sickness, experienced an "early kick," or "look different" from the way they looked before the birth of a daughter. Even the wheat and barley urine test introduced in 1350 B.C. has reappeared periodically. Early in this century researchers claimed that it actually did work, although subsequent evaluations did not confirm their optimistic findings.

Sex Determination "Recipes" of the Past

The combination of widespread misunderstanding about human reproduction and a fervent desire to control sex outcome has led to the development of hundreds of theories on the "how to" of sex preselection.

As you can tell from the list of references in the back of this book, just about every generation has had its own theory, and at least one book that elaborated on it. The sex predetermination books of the 1800s and early 1900s make especially fascinating reading. They have elaborate, authoritative-sounding titles that offer something for everyone. One thing they do not have is modesty on the part of the author. Most of these books were privately printed and begin with a fanfare on the theme, "At last, at last I have the answer!" And of course a few years later each of them was replaced by another book, often one that offered exactly opposite advice.

Some of the methods advocated were pure superstition, and no serious efforts were made to prove their effectiveness. For instance, an ancient Swedish custom called for the bride to sleep with a baby boy on the night prior to her nuptials so that she would be ensured a son as her first born. The Yugoslavs were less specific, recommending merely a young boy. Toward the same end, other cultures arranged for young boys to leap into the saddle when a bride first dismounts from her mule at her husband's house. In many countries a man desiring a son is still commonly advised to have intercourse with his boots on; in others, it's evidently thought that a hat works better than boots.

The legends of Austria were somehow entangled ·
with nut trees. In some areas, the midwife would bury
the placenta under a nut tree to ensure that the next
child to arrive would be male. In other parts of the
country, peasants believed that a good year in the crop
of nuts foretold a good year in the crop of baby boys.
The natives of West Bengal in Africa believed that
intercourse on even-numbered days would produce a
male, on odd-numbered days a female; but it is doubt-
ful that this premise could have endured for very long
without someone becoming suspicious.

No more reliable, however, are those methods based
on the pseudoscience of astrology. For instance, the
editor of the *American Physician,* Frank Kraft, M.D.,
in 1908 (in *Sex of Offspring: A Modern Discovery of a
Primeval Law*), and Thomas Reed, M.D., in 1913 *(Sex:
Its Origin and Determination),* inform us that the timing of sexual intercourse in relation to the moon's
phases is the all-important factor; specifically, that if
coitus takes place at or near the middle of the "positive" phases of the sex or tide cycle, a male is the
result, while at or near the middle of the "negative" or
passive phase, a female is conceived. A book in our
own time (1973), *Natural Birth Control and How to
Choose the Sex of Your Child,* updates us on the current happenings in the field of astrological birth control
and sex selection techniques. According to the authors, Sheila Ostrander and Lynn Schroeder, the position of the moon in the skies at the time of conception
determines the sex of the child: "For instance, if the
moon is in the sign of Aries, Gemini, Leo, Libra,
Sagittarius or Aquarius at the time of the mother's
lunar birthday (at the time of ovulation), then the child
conceived at that time will be a boy. If the moon is in
the sign of Taurus, Cancer, Virgo, Scorpio, Capricorn

or Pisces when the sun/moon angle recurs, the child conceived would be a girl." To find out what sign the moon is in on a particular date, these two would-be sex determinationists suggested that couples consult an "ephemeris," a set of tables listing the locations in the zodiac of the solar system bodies on each day of the year. All you needed for these recipes was a clock, an almanac, and, of course, the authors' book.

Many other methods have been given serious scientific attention at some point in history. In particular, six categories of sex determination techniques have been particularly resilient over the years, those that claim the child's sex is a function of either (1) the side of the body in which he or she originated; (2) the relative strength of the parents; (3) the parental diet; (4) autosuggestion and psychological stimuli; (5) the timing of insemination within the menstrual cycle; or (6) the chemical state of the female reproductive tract just before and during intercourse.

For reasons discussed below, the first four methods are no longer in the running for the ultimate prize of human sex control. Since the last two areas—timing of insemination and vaginal chemistry—are still quite relevant, we will discuss them in detail in later chapters.

ALTERNATING CURRENTS: THOSE RIGHT AND LEFT THEORIES

There are two sides of the human body. Perhaps males come from one side, females from the other? Well, you can see why people would at least give the idea some consideration.

In the absence of any other suggestion, this theory looked pretty good to ancient and some not-so-ancient medical researchers. The question of which sex to assign to which side probably never came up: it seemed obvious that the "superior" of the two sexes would emanate from the allegedly more developed and warmer of the two sides—the right. (Since right-handedness was traditionally associated with justice and strength, while left-handedness represented weakness and evil, it's apparent which of the sexes was responsible for the designation.)

Hippocrates taught that "the male fetus is usually seated in the right, the female in the left side of the uterus." Assuming that the uterus was duplex and extending the logic to further assume that the right testicle would emit a "male seed," eager prospective fathers would tie strings around their right testicles in an effort to stimulate production, and then position themselves and their wives so that the male seed had a good chance of entering the male side of the uterine chamber. It is hardly necessary to add that these must have been couples who took the sex determination issue very seriously. If after all these acrobatic maneuvers a son did not appear, well, it must be the woman's fault, or so many enraged and unenlightened new fathers probably concluded. Apparently the more suspicious among them reached the eventual deduction that perhaps they were tying up the wrong side—that a tight string around the *left* testicle would seal the exit from the female seed factory. So at various times in history, men dedicated to their task settled on tying the left side instead.

The learned Aristotle must have been deeply intrigued by the human reproductive process, given that he devoted so much attention to it in his writings. While opposed to the "string" technique, or perhaps merely confused by it, he did have a wealth of advice to offer. Among other proclamations that we will get to in the coming pages, he recommended that the woman should lie on her right side after intercourse "in order that this side might be the place of conception, for therein is the greatest generation of heat, which is the chief procuring cause of male children." Chances of success were said to improve if she kept warm and "with little motion," presumably so that the sperm wouldn't be tempted to wander off.

In some circles the string was abandoned in favor of the more convenient, and no less effective, method of simple pinching—the right testicle for a boy, the left for a girl. Centuries later, in the eighteenth to be exact, French noblemen who were also opposed to all this tying and pinching evolved yet another technique: those frevently desiring a male heir simply had their left testicle removed entirely. When approximately 50 percent of the offspring turned out to be girls, the obvious assumption was that the surgeon must have left behind a small amount of female-bearing tissue.

The right-left theory survived through many centuries in at least one of its various forms. An 1870 issue of the British medical journal *Lancet* carried a letter that stated, "From many inquiries I have made among my married friends, I have no hesitation in saying that when men are in the habit of sleeping on the right side of their wives, they beget male children and when on the left, female." Was the writer serious? His comments engendered enough positive responses from the medical community to indicate that some of his colleagues certainly took them seriously.

Whether through lack of originality or sheer desperation, as recently as 1958 (and possibly still) one version of the right-left theory was still practiced in parts of rural India. Here—more than 2,000 years after the proposals of Hippocrates and Aristotle—it was the wife's duty to grab and squeeze her husband's left testicle at the exact moment of ejaculation so that only the right, i.e. male, sperm would enter. If subsequently a daughter was born, the unfortunate lady was beaten for not squeezing hard enough. The consequences of squeezing *too* hard appear to have gone unrecorded, perhaps because they were unprintable.

Far less painful, if just as useless, is yet another widespread "boy" custom that lingers on in the backwoods of Pennsylvania and many parts of the South, perhaps other locales as well. This one has the prospective father hanging his trousers over the right bedpost before he sets about the business of begetting. (It is well that, unlike boots and hat, it is not customary to wear the trousers to bed.)

The heyday of the right-left philosophy was in the early part of this century, when Dr. Ernest Rumley Dawson, a member of the Council of the Obstetrical Society of London and a Fellow of the Royal Society of Medicine, announced confidently that "boy eggs" were released from the right ovary and "girl eggs" from the left. He explained that there were exactly thirteen ovulations a year, and that the ovaries alternated. Although you'd be unable to choose the sex of your first child because you'd have no idea which ovary was operative in the month of conception, you would, if you kept careful menstrual histories, be able to choose the sex of the children who followed. Dawson added some more helpful advice: first, if you wanted a boy baby, the wife should avoid horseback riding, as it might cause a cramp in her right ovary; second, during sexual intercourse the wife should lie on the side, left or right, whose ovary she wanted to favor.

Dr. Dawson was absolutely positive that he was correct, and because of his professional credentials he engendered a greal deal of enthusiasm among his patients and some laymen who heard about his theory. One follower, Mrs. Laura A. Calhoun, was enthusiastic enough about the Dawson right-left ovary theory to write a book (*The Law of Sex Determination and Its Practical Application*) about it in 1910, wherein she added for good measure her personal belief that there were also right and left sperm. She explained the details of implementing the formula, using, of course, the most impeccably ladylike language.

The medical profession was less receptive to the Dawson idea about alternating ovaries. Colleagues pointed out that Dawson's theory failed to explain how some women who had had a right ovary removed still had male children. But Dawson had an answer for that too: the surgeon must have inadvertently left a little bit of the right ovary behind.

The case of Dr. Dawson presents an illustrious example of what happens when the sex predetermination mania takes over and rational, scientific evaluation becomes impossible. Despite all the evidence to the contrary, he was to defend his theory to the grave. A few years before his death he formally presented his concepts in a book, *The Causation of Sex in Man,* dedicated to a "medical martyr," Ignatius Semmelweiss, who years before had been ridiculed by his peers for presenting the theory that hospital-based infections were responsible for mothers' deaths in maternity wards, an idea that was later confirmed. Dr. Dawson's dedication referred to Semmelweiss as a man who was "disbelieved, despised, and ridiculed by his colleagues and teachers, finally dying insane, a victim of the relentless persecution and contemptuous opposition to which he was subjected. . . . There is nothing more thankless than the attempt to influence a field of public opinion." Dawson thought that he, like Semmelweiss, would be a hero someday. And so did his wife. When Dawson died in 1921 his widow reissued his book. "I share my husband's confidence," she wrote, "that advancing science will one day establish the truth of the position which this book seeks to explain."

The Dawsons were just two of many victims of enthusiasm without benefit of facts. Today, contrary to what you may read in some sex selection books, we know that the ovaries do *not* necessarily alternate in releasing eggs from month to month, and that it is the male sperm, not the egg, which determines the sex of the child.

PARENTAL STRENGTH

The notion that the relative strength or mental attributes of the husband and wife might have an influence on the sex of their child has been around for centuries, but it was given special attention during the nineteenth and early twentieth centuries. This theory is somewhat confusing because there are two conflicting versions of it.

If you were to hypothesize that parental strength was the key, you might initially assume that it would be the stronger parent who would determine the sex of the child. That is, if the father were big and strong and masculine, perhaps the odds on a son would be greater. Hippocrates went along with this, explaining that the relative quantity and strength of the "male and female semen" determined sex. Male semen by definition was stronger, unless there wasn't enough of it, in which case it would be "overwhelmed by an abundance of the weaker." In the Babylonian Talmud, Jewish folklore postulated that the baby's gender depended on which parent was more passionate at conception, which must have generated some interesting bedroom dialogues.

Intrigued by this "dominance" philosophy, Aristotle expanded it to proclaim that strength and vigor were affected by the weather. "More males are born if copulation takes place when a north wind rather than a south wind blows," he wrote, "for the south wind is moister." Besides wind direction and phases of the moon, other would-be scholars, then and since, have attributed the sex ratio to rainfall, temperature, and other climatic conditions. A relatively recent study by an Illinois doctor concluded that more females are conceived in "warm weather" (whatever that means) and vice versa. Considering the variables involved, the significance of such alleged findings remains obscure other than its apparent attempt to support the notion that the "stronger sex" can be expected to triumph in the face of adversity.

Nevertheless, the temperature myth has been increasing in popularity since 1979 when a pair of researchers released the news that the sex of sea turtles is directly related to temperature. Eggs incubated in captivity must be held at a specific optimum temperature in order to maintain a more or less balanced sex ratio. Two degrees higher produces all females, two degrees lower all males. (In their natural habitat the problem does not exist because of daily fluctuations in the temperature of the beach sand where the eggs are laid.) Since sea turtles and humans have so little in common in other respects, the discovery seems to have little relevance for higher forms of life.

In 1926, Nils O. Lundell, M.D., felt strongly enough about the weaker-stronger theory to swear to his method before a Nassau County, New York, notary public. Dr. Lundell identified the "strength of the blood" as the key to sex control and prescribed "tonics, foods, fresh air and rest" for men who wanted sons.

Edward Carr, in his 1938 book, *Choosing the Sex of Children: How to Decide in Advance of Conception Whether One's Offspring Shall Be Male or Female, How to Avoid Having Effeminate Boys or Masculine Girls,* agreed; the stronger parent was responsible for the outcome, he said; every male sperm strives to produce a male, and a "girl's life originates in the full flame of mother power." The practical advice here was to have sex when the wife was weak and tired if you wanted a boy.

This version of the parental-strength recipe was revived again in 1951 by M. B. Abboud in *Love, Life and Truth,* whose readers learned that a woman who wanted sons should eat less and lift twenty- to thirty-pound weights each day until she was completely exhausted.

Considering the mystery that surrounded the topic of human reproduction, it is understandable why the stronger-parent theory became popular. But what is perplexing is that the "superior opposites" theory—that is, the claim that the child's sex is the *opposite* of that of the stronger parent—was infinitely *more* popular. We can only assume it most likely began as a "sour grapes" rationale that bloomed into a full-scale explanation of why the superior-same idea so often failed.

George B. Starkweather, a late-nineteenth-century writer, was probably the most vocal advocate of the superior-opposites school of sex predetermination, elaborating on a theory that had been advanced some fifty years before.

And, of course, Mr. Starkweather had a book too, one with a particularly handsome title: *The Law of Sex: Being an Exposition of the Natural Laws by Which the Sex of Offspring Is Controlled in Man And The Lower Animals: And Giving The Solution to Various Social Problems.* In this volume, which begins with the announcement that he is making known "a new discovery of a great law of nature," Starkweather castigates other authors for indulging in wild speculation and then goes to great lengths to define "superiority," basing most of his categorizations on temperament, will power, complexion, shape of head, eye and hair color, and shape of the nose, mouth, and chin. Here are a few passages from this extraordinary book:

. . . reproductive function gives vigour and tone to the whole frame and, if kept under proper restraint, is conducive to "superiority." . . .

I say that a person with poor digestion is generally "superior" to one whose digestion is remarkably good . . .

A prominent nose is in itself an excellent feature and generally denotes a person ready for great enterprises and achievements, just as surely as a flat nose betokens an ease-loving lymphatic nature.

Starkweather included illustrations and descriptions of some model couples. With regard to the first couple shown, named A1 and B1, he writes:

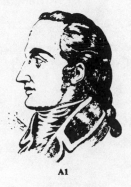
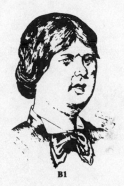

A1   B1

A1 is a model figure of a man. It is hardly necessary to discuss the different features of that noble
face for they are one and all perfect. There are
doubtless lower types of womanhood than B1 but
they are difficult to find: everything about her is
gross and repulsive. Assuming it to be possible
that such a man could ever marry such a woman,
what would be the sex of the issue? . . . Were they
to have twenty children, every one would most
surely be a girl.

The second couple, A20 and B20 (next page), is,
Starkweather feels, an example of the other extreme.
They would inevitably have sons, who, by a fortunate
extension of Starkweather's ideas, would take after the
mother rather than the father.

But if you are a man with a nose of less than desirable stature, and you want a daughter, there is hope.
You have two choices. You can build yourself up, if
only temporarily, so that you engender the opposite
sex (Starkweather recommended Turkish baths). Or

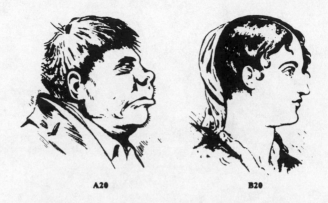

A20   B20

you can do something to displace your wife from her
pedestal of superiority (rape is recommended here because it "lowers a woman's superiority").

Samuel Hough Terry was another believer in the
superior-opposites theory. And, yes, he had a book
too: *Controlling Sex in Generation: The Physical Law
Influencing The Embryo of Man and Brute And Its
Direction To Produce Male or Female Offspring At
Will,* published in 1885. (This book was so popular that
it was reissued in 1917 under the happier title *The
Secret of Sex.*) Terry offered a wide variety of "evidence" to show that the sex of the resulting baby was
always the opposite of that of the parent who was
stronger at the time of coitus. Wives of farmers, he
points out, because they are robust and healthy, have
more sons than city ladies do. Wives brought up reli-
giously are, by definition, weak and passive and "prone
to think about death more frequently" and thus inevitably will have more daughters. If you want a son, Terry
advises bridegrooms, be sure to pick your bride carefully. And he is specific: she should be five feet to five

feet ten, should measure *at least* (emphasis his) thirty-six inches around the bust and have "sufficient strength to readily put up a 25-pound dumbbell in each hand . . . and to take a five-mile walk out and back every day without special fatigue." On the other hand, if you want a daughter, the father should build himself up. "Any boy can beget a boy," he warns, "but it takes a man to beget a girl."

Terry offered a case history which he felt described the ideal circumstances for the conception of a male child, the point being that if a woman gets sexually excited and charged with "electricity," she'll have a son. The story concerns a young woman being sued for divorce who explained to the court that she had been seduced against her will. "Being in the young man's chamber early one morning on some household errand, he grasped her by the hand and straightaway such a thrill went through her whole body that she had no control over herself." And (much to her husband's chagrin) she had a boy.

Nineteen-sixteen was a big year for the superior-opposites theory. Two separate publications appeared, *Natural Painless Childbirth and the Art of Sex Determination,* by Filip Sylvan, and *Within the Bud: Procreation of a Healthy, Happy and Beautiful Child of the Desired Sex,* by Louis Dechmann. Sylvan's advice was simple: a woman wanting a son was to increase her "constitutional strength," while making sure that her husband avoided all types of exercise for at least five months prior to the planned conception.

Dechmann's advice was much more complicated. As he explained to the *New York Times,* he had "at last wrested from nature one of her intrinsic secrets after many years of study," and had identified (and taken

out a copyright on) the "laws of latent reserve energy."
His idea was that the egg and sperm struggle for control, the victory going to the seed which is weakest at
the moment of conception. Dechmann believed that
the weaker cell eventually becomes dominant through
the force of its "latent reserve energy." In other words,
if the wife took steps to make herself weak and tired,
and intercourse took place at a time in the menstrual
cycle when the egg had lost its "strength," the weaker
cell would "win," and the result would be a boy who
looked like his mother.

The superior-opposites theory did not fade away
with Dechmann and Sylvan. In 1925 it was revived by
William Roscoe Tucker in his best-selling book, *Do
You Wish to Choose the Sex of Your Children? A
Lecture on the Subject of Sex Control in Man,* which
made another contribution to the growing "evidence"
that the sex of the child was always opposite that of the
stronger parent. According to Tucker, the children of
female farm laborers born in December, January, and
February were usually girls. Why? Because the children were conceived in March, April, and May, a time
of the year when the women worked very hard and
were too tired and weak to conceive a boy.

As late as 1960, Chyan-Tzaw Wang, in a book
pulished in Taiwan and entitled *Human Sex Control,*
informed his readers that he was introducing "a new
yet perfect mechanism of human sex control to the
world," and proceeded to restate the superior-opposites theory. Statistical evidence to support his contention included the observation that fat men married
to thin women have more girls and that old men and
young women have boys. If a wife can only arrange to
be young and put on a little weight to gain strength,
she'll be sure to present her husband with a boy baby.

YOUR BABY IS WHAT YOU EAT

The idea that diet influences sex outcome is as old as our earliest medical records. Male-producing pre-love-making apéritifs included animal blood, raisin and other types of wine, raw vinegar, the testes of various animals, salted fish and meats, and leaves cooked in olive oil and salt. In ancient Rome plain lettuce was the popular food. In parts of Africa, oysters (unsalted!) were the going thing for a girl—a myth that still pops up occasionally—while folk recipes in most of the rest of the world called for sweets. "Boy foods" included, at one time or another, almost anything that was bitter, sour, or salty.

Aristotle proposed a male concoction of wine and herbs for all those women carefully lying on their right sides with little motion. Macabre rites during the Middle Ages specified a meal of red meat and gruesome brews of wine and lion's blood, after which the pair copulated under a full moon while the local abbot prayed. Whenever the ritual produced a daughter, there was a simple explanation: an untimely cloud must have passed across the moon at the inopportune moment.

Some superstitions were content to leave the wine straight and preferably consumed in quantity, which appears to have had something to do with weakening the appropriate partner. Napoleon, writing to his pregnant goddaughter, advised her that she could ensure a male birth by drinking pure wine daily during her confinement. (In due course, and despite the fact that she followed his advice, she delivered a fine daughter.) Nevertheless, sipping wine was surely more pleasurable than what the followers of one later scientist had to endure: They were told to drink periodic doses of baking soda.

It was Dr. Leopold Schenk, Director of the Embryological Institute in Vienna, who in 1898 was probably the first scholar to officially set forth the idea that the sex of the child was directly related to what mother ate before and during the pregnancy. Naturally he wrote a book, *The Determination of Sex,* in which he confidently proclaimed that he had "snatched a secret from Nature," the precious secret being that "the nutrition of the mother plays a leading part in the development of the ovum within her body." His advice, really not much more than an expansion of the old folk tales, sounds like a cross between one of our "new, modern, revolutionary, guaranteed weight-loss diets" and a nursery rhyme: women who wanted sons were to go on a high-protein, low-carbohydrate diet; those who wanted daughters could eat all they wanted from the food category "sugar and spice and everything nice." His patients were to evaluate their progress by means of daily urine tests.

The philosophy behind Schenk's miracle male-producing diet was that a high-protein menu would weaken the mother (anyone who's been on a low-carbohydrate diet understands this), but would simultaneously lead to the development of a male-producing ovum. Since males were superior physically before as well as after birth, they could survive this nutritional strain and would simply absorb all the protein. Weak little girl babies could not. (Evidently the daughter of the Empress of Russia at that time remained unaware of this phenomenon. She insisted on being born a girl in spite of her mother's strict adherence to Schenk's diet.)

In 1908 Dr. Frank Kraft reinforced the belief that good nutrition leads to the preponderance of female infants in *Sex of Offspring: A Modern Discovery of Primeval Law.* In addition to his studies of astrological influences, Dr. Kraft reported that more boys were born after cholera epidemics and wars and during the colder months, since "the female has not the strength to endure the continual strain and adverse conditions."

A sex determination theory is never quite established until someone comes up with exactly the opposite advice. Percy John McElrath did this for Dr. Kraft's idea in his authoritative-sounding volume, *The Key to Sex Control or the Cellular Determination of Sex and the Physiological Laws Which Govern Its Control,* published in 1911. McElrath's "how to have a son" advice is to eat well, because good maternal nutrition will lead to rapid ovum growth and an increased chance of fertilizing a fresh, mature cell, which would by definition be male. Thus wives were to eat meats and fats and a moderate amount of carbohydrates. Husbands hoping for sons were to focus on a high-carbohydrate diet so that "sperm are produced more slowly, and there is a tendency to the elaboration of the best specimens in both size and quality." (Gardeners familiar with the process of disbudding will understand how McElrath might have arrived at this notion.)

As the 20th century unfolded, nutritional nonsense invaded the area of baby production just as it has invaded every other aspect of our lives. The difference today is that so much of the dietary misadvice is being advocated by professional people who ought to know better in light of medical advances in the past half-century. But they persist, often dredging up some of the old folklore to support their theories.

Just a few years ago, Dr. Joseph Stolkowski of the Université Pierre et Marie Curie in Paris became smitten with texts from the "distant past" indicating that sex distribution of cows and sheep was related to their diets in the pasture. Fanning the flames was another

study that claimed "marked changes" (without spec-
ifying what they were) in the sex ratio of rabbits fed
liquid supplements of glucose, glycine (a protein deriv-
ative), and ascorbic acid (vitamin C). Stolkowski set
about conducting his own experiments, later joined by
Dr. Jacques Lorrain of the Hôpital du Sacré-Coeur in
Montreal. Couched in a great deal of gobbledygook
about pH values, osmotic pressure, and ion exchange,
the formulae are basically concerned with mineral intake. According to their somewhat limited research, it
all has to do with the ratio of potassium plus sodium to
the amount of calcium plus magnesium. A high ratio,
particularly as it applies to potassium, will produce a
boy, they declare; low ratios (especially in the amount
of potassium) a girl.

Stolkowski and Lorrain maintained that their dietary
method resulted in an 80 percent success rate for the
desired sex, but their claim as reported in the *International Journal of Gynecology and Obstetrics* (1980)
leaves many unanswered questions. Remember, we're
starting out with an approximate 50 percent success
rate by doing nothing at all, with a plus-or-minus additional number based on mere chance, particularly when
so relatively few couples (260) were studied. No mention is made of such important variables as timing of
intercourse, and the only apparent control group seems
to have been the population at large.

To uncover a solution to the boy-girl puzzle as simple
as diet control would be wondrous indeed. Unfortunately, the data in this case only support the theory
to the extent that one wishes to interpret them that
way. In other words, they've led us no further ahead in
the realm of sex selection than we were in the days of
salted fish and oysters.

Undaunted, the theory could not be laid to rest without a book about it. In 1982, Sally Langendoen and William Proctor put together *The Pre-Conception Gender Diet* (they should have named it The *Mis*conception Gender Diet), about half of which consists of recipes and menus. Basically it adheres to the same Stolkowski/Lorrain tenets of high-protein, high-salt, low-calcium, and an abundance of potassium for a boy; and, of course, exactly the opposite for a girl. At least the authors are conscientious enough to include a number of caveats for prospective parents who might be susceptible to extremely high levels of salt (especially victims of high blood pressure), and to either high or low levels of calcium. What they do *not* mention is the inherent danger of any faddish diet, *especially* when pregnancy is imminent. At a time when obstetricians and other health professionals everywhere are promoting the importance of superior nutrition *before* pregnancy (as well as during), along comes a book rousing its readers to try a distinctly *un*balanced diet on the off-chance that they may be able to manipulate the sexual outcome of their anticipated child.

Husbands are advised to join their dieting wives, primarily to provide "moral support." The regimen, we're told, should be started four to six weeks before attempting conception and discontinued as soon as pregnancy is confirmed—or after six months, whichever comes first. Chances are that only the most determined could hold out that long.

The boy diet excludes all dairy products but is very big on salty meats, pork products and dried fruits. The girl diet calls for salt-free everything and vitamin C supplements in place of citrus fruits. No alcoholic beverages are allowed (girls only) and a maximum of only eight ounces of any carbonated beverage (that's two-thirds of an average can). Both diets are skimpy on raw greens and fruits, especially the girl menus which are generally opposed to raw anything. The chief virtue seems to be that both regimens are relatively low-calorie, at approximately 1,800 per day. Evidently the authors assume that all prospective parents like to camp out in the kitchen: the menus are rather more complicated than most of us are interested in eating, much less preparing three times a day. Further, for a girl they recommend many homemade recipes (such as apple pie) because the commercial varieties tend to be higher in salt.

Beyond the obvious shortcomings, the diets are something of a puzzle. Langendoen and Proctor tell us that the boy prescription contains approximately 5,000 mg/day of sodium, which isn't harmful because it's "well within the usual daily consumption of 2,000–6,000 mg/day." Actually, most estimates place the figure even higher than that. So what this amounts to is that the "high-salt" boy-diet is no higher, and possibly lower, than the amounts ordinarily consumed anyway—assuming, of course, that the 5,000 mg they cite is accurate.

Even more confusing is the girl-diet ban on citrus products. At first thought it would seem this is because citrus is a good source of potassium; yet potato, which is an even better source of potassium, is included almost every day. (Other elements in those two foods are roughly comparable, although oranges contain a fair amount of calcium, which should only serve to strengthen its case as a "girl" food, yet they are not allowed.)

The *Gender Diet* further presents an array of tidbits that, although not necessarily incorrect, are distinctly misleading. The authors cite insignificant studies in support of their case without pointing out the insignificance; they note that Japan has a sex ratio at birth of 106.4 boys for every 100 girls (compared to the U.S. rate of 105:100) thereby implying that the Japanese diet must be more boy-oriented (i.e., salty); and they defend the old wine-for-a-boy myths by pointing out that wine contains a substantial amount of potassium. (So do a large variety of foods commonly included in the average American diet.)

Although statements are made several times that diet does influence sex, the authors admit they don't know why. The "why" is supposed to be unimportant anyway, since they deny they are advocating any "radical" eating changes. No dairy products for up to six months is radical.

Regrettably, in the rampant pursuit of nutritional misinformation that is so much a part of the American scene these days, there will be some couples who will believe, and who will attempt to follow the program. This in spite of the fact that the past few years of carefully conducted research has uncovered a direct relationship between a woman's pre-pregnancy diet and the health of her baby (whether boy or girl). Obviously, this means that from the moment she even thinks about a baby, she should strive to maintain balanced eating habits. For anyone to propose otherwise is unconscionable.

IT'S ALL IN YOUR MIND

The sex of unborn offspring is not influenced by right and left orientations, nutrition or any other physical factors. It's all in your mind. By concentrating on thoughts of your goal, you can do whatever you want. And that includes choosing the sex of your child. So goes the advice of the autosuggestion school of thought.

Aristotle was convinced that imagination had a great deal to do with determining a baby's sex. While those ladies who desired boys reclined on their right sides sipping herbal wines, those opting for girls were to lie on their left sides and think strongly of a female. Other superstitions had women dressing in men's clothing before intercourse, or chanting themselves into a state of near-hypnosis as they concentrated heavily on the sex of their choice.

But it was not until 1899 that C. Wilbur Taber wrote the classic book in this area, *Suggestion: The Secret of Sex,* emphasizing the premise that "the determination of sex lies within the volition of every individual." He also had a pinch of the "parental strength theory" mixed into his recipe: that the woman should be weak, indeed passive, during the sex act to ensure a son. His advice is worth quoting:

> There should be thorough preparation for the event, months before the procreation takes place . . . and when the procreative act takes place, it should be with one thought in mind . . . It might be well before procreation takes place to practice how to become passive. Have the wife recline in an easy position, free from all tension or mental anxiety and making long passes from her head to her feet, suggest a quiet restful sleep. Continue such suggestions until she becomes entirely passive or drops into a light sleep. Then, without disturbing her, place your hand on her forehead

and gently rubbing her head, give her support that the desired result will be secured . . .

Talk in a quiet tone, telling her that it is possible to regulate the sex of one's child if desired. . . . Tell her that the next child will be a son.

In summary, put your wife to sleep and then sneak up on her ("without disturbing her"). Taber adds that once the "procreative act" has taken place under these desirable circumstances, husbands should read their wives bedtime stories, choosing from biographies of men who became famous.

W. Wallace Hoffman, M.D., agreed that sex outcome was a direct function of the mind's ability to control the body. His 1916 book, *Sterility and Choice of Sex in the Human Family: A Subject With Which Medical Books Do Not Deal, Having Special Reference To The Causes of Change In And The Theories of Determination Of Sex In The Unborn Together With A Little Thought On The Question Of Sterility,* relates a series of stories about the effects of the spirit on the body. One concerns a young lady who witnessed a trolley wire catch on fire in London. Although she was not hurt, she immediately fell dead because "she simply thought she was in danger and thought so intensely that something gave way and separated her spirit from her body." Just as this woman could convince herself that she was going to die, others can use that mind power to conceive a child of the sex they desire. To Hoffman and his supporters, it was no surprise that more males seemed to be born during and just after wars, since "men and women (were) devoting their minds to the question of male children to replace the ones eliminated."

Not only could a couple's thoughts at the moment of

conception influence the sex of the child, but Hoffman grimly warned that the couple's state of mind would be directly transferred to the child they were creating. Thus even a habitually sober person who has a couple of highballs before he goes to bed could be asking for trouble, since inebriation raises the risk of begetting "epileptic, paralytic, idiotic and insane children . . . with marked weakness of the mind. . . . A single embrace given in a moment of drunkenness may be fatal to an entire generation."

A great enthusiast of the Hoffman mind-over-matter theory was Cary S. Cox, author of *Causes and Control of Sex* (1923). Cox had stories of his own to add to the case of mind control: a fisherman's wife was once frightened by a turtle. Her child was therefore born with flippers instead of feet. Cox referred anyone who didn't believe the story to the Boston Museum, where, he explained, the turtle-child was preserved in alcohol. If one woman could produce a turtle-baby, another could certain choose male or female. Cox advised that staring at portraits of male children was very helpful.

Related to the autosuggestion theories of sex control are claims that outside psychological forces can have an effect on a baby's sex. Researchers through the ages have suggested that stress is an important factor, the sex of the child being the same as that of the less-stressed sexual partner. In the early 1960s there were reports that pilots of fighter aircraft had more than their share of girl children when they returned home, and the explanation offered was that stress might inhibit male births, perhaps through a physical mechanism such as raising the body temperature to the point where male-producing sperm are killed or incapacitated.

An Iowa State research team at one point was looking into the possibility that stress is an important variable, noting that anxious fathers tend to produce a female child, anxious mothers a male. (There is no comment about what happens when they are *both* anxious.) A stressed father is one who "is striving to get ahead on the job or in life. The stressed mother is a social climber, a career woman, or merely homesick." In a 1974 article in the *Journal of Genetic Psychology* we encounter another variation of the stress-sex theory. The *Journal* reported a study of ten raped women, nine of whom had sons (noting that the one woman who had a daughter had had a previous relationship with the man involved), the conclusion being that perhaps stressed women (as in the rape situation) would be more likely to have sons.

The stress theories are interesting but so far have little, if any, foundation. Studies of a few fighter pilots and ten rape victims do not make scientific facts.

THE ULTIMATE IN SEX DETERMINATION THEORIES

If a prize were given to the author with the most original sex predetermination prescription, it would have to go to Francis Buzzacott, author of *Mystery of the Sexes: Secrets of Past and Future Human Creationism,* published in 1914. You know his book is going to be different as soon as you open it and find that it begins with a quotation from himself:

> When true philosophy begs to be heard, the
> Wise and Incredulous Oft Refuse to Listen.

> Buzzacott

Mr. Buzzacott's key to sex determination is abstinence from sexual intercourse, his premise being that nature never meant us to be divided into males and females in the first place. It was "by persistent sexual intercourse, incestuous conduct, evil thought, deed, they both fell, became twain, separated, disunited, differentiated." We are advised to avoid coitus: "sexual intercourse is a crime against the body and will yet be so declared. Christ himself taught pure love was not passion." Instead, we should reproduce "normally" ("the male is not an absolute necessity in procreation"), and eventually, according to Buzzacott, we will all return to our natural hermaphrodite state and never have to worry about choosing the sex of children.

Amazed if not enlightened, we can now turn our attention from the ingenious theories of the past to modern-day knowledge of the biology of human reproduction. The accumulation of knowledge in this area has been a painfully slow process. Nature's mysteries are not easily solved. But we do have a great deal of information on reproductive physiology, and these facts provide the essential building blocks in our quest to choose in advance the sex of unborn children.

Patented Sept. 5, 1922.   1,428,065

UNITED STATES PATENT OFFICE.

HUBERT ROYDS TIDSWELL, OF WINNINGTON, ENGLAND.
SEX CALCULATOR.

Application filed March 30, 1920. Serial No. 369,927.

To all whom it may concern:

Be it known that I, HUBERT ROYDS TIDSWELL, a subject of the King of Great Britain and Ireland, residing at 46 Win-
5 nington Lane, Winnington, Cheshire, England, have invented certain new and useful Improvements in Sex Calculators, and I do hereby declare the following to be a full, clear, and exact description of the in-
10 vention, such as will enable others skilled in the art to which it appertains to make and use the same.

A device for finding the sex of all children, born to the same woman, after the
15 first child has been born, when one knows the approximate dates of births of the expected children and the sex of the child previously born. The device also shows when fertilization must take place for a
20 particular sex to be born.

This invention is based on the well-known and proved theory that in normal women the ovaries ovulate alternately, and that one ovary always produces male
25 ova and the other female ova, and that this action occurs at regular intervals, the sequence not being disturbed by gestation or lactation. Consequently if the date of birth and sex of first child born be known,
30 one can predict or determine the sex of subsequent children. The device consists of two or more parts of any regular geometrical form, and

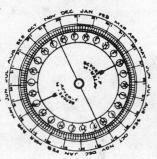

PATENT OFFICE HAS ACCEPTED "SEX-DETERMINATION"

That "the well known and proved theory" on which this calculator is based is a proven fallacy has not prevented this inventor from displaying considerable ingenuity in the development of this device. It is not difficult to cite instances of women with only one ovary producing children of both sexes, and reference may also be made to the birds, which consistently produce the sexes in approximately equal numbers with only one functional ovary.

Reprinted with permission of the *Journal of Heredity*.

3

How Babies Are Made (Advanced Course)

There are many "sex books" on the market today that claim to offer you everything you ever wanted to know and more. For better or worse, the same material that a generation or so ago was primarily available only in a "plain brown wrapper" is now out of the closet onto the shelves. The expanding social permissiveness of the 1970s and 1980s was evidently perceived by a host of would-be "experts" as an open invitation to grind out his/her personal approach to the subject. As with most how-to manuals, some are considerably better than others.

The majority of lay people—and a large proportion of medical and public health professionals—know a great deal more about the bizarre aspects of human sexuality than they do about the basic facts of the menstrual cycle, the conditions under which conception can occur, the physiology of pregnancy, and the factors that determine whether a baby will be a boy or a girl.

For example, during the early 1970s I conducted a study of sex and reproduction knowledge in a sample of nurses, social workers, and high-school teachers and found that over 80 percent of them could not correctly identify the days of the menstrual cycle when conception was most likely to occur. Ninety percent of the people were unable to answer the most basic questions about the male reproductive system. These dismal findings reflected a serious gap in professional education, and as a result I prepared (under the sponsorship of Syntex Laboratories) a nationwide programmed learning course, entitled quite basically *Human Reproduction and Family Planning*, to teach health professionals, the very group of people who have the responsibility for teaching others, the elementary "facts of life."

With the arrival of the mid-1980s, I am heartened to learn that an increasing number of schools now routinely include reproductive physiology (however cursory) as part of their curriculum. On the other hand, I find it frustrating that so many others still do not allow the subject to be taught, and of those that do, most require written permission from the parents. Such attitudes imply that reproduction is somehow unnatural or of less biological importance than digestion or respiration.

While most couples today (although by no means all) are well-versed in the procedure for "making babies," along with a smattering of other knowledge, the fact remains that the majority do not really have much

understanding of the actual events that may or may not
lead to pregnancy. As in the course I designed, I am
here going to present the basics, admittedly in a somewhat "kneebone is connected to the thighbone" style,
but in a far more detailed way than most general sex
manuals.

If you have little technical background, the various
segments may at first seem complicated and the termi-
nology unfamiliar, and I realize you may even be
tempted to skip this chapter entirely. I urge you to give
it a try. Read it slowly if necessary (you're not being
timed), study the diagrams, and reread anything that
seems unclear. You will most likely discover the material to be no more complex than a great many other
topics you deal with on a more regular basis. You may
even feel you should be awarded a Ph.D. in reproductive physiology by the time you finish it, but I have two
specific reasons for including this material in our overall discussion of sex predetermination.

First, I feel that you must understand the complexities of the reproductive cycle if you are to be successful in implementing my recommendations for
increasing your odds of having a child of the sex of
your choice. As you'll learn in the next chapter, the key
lies in predicting the day of ovulation, the release of the
ovum or egg from the ovary. In order to do this you
must have an awareness of the female sex hormones
and body structures involved in reproduction and the
methods of self-observation that will help you predict
the critical reproductive events.

Second, I am offering this detailed account of the
events leading to conception and birth as an antidote to
what I feel is a very unfortunate side effect of the
"contraceptive revolution." Many people have come to

take childbearing for granted, referring to a baby as if he or she were a commodity, one they may or may not need any more of today. I've encountered more than one individual whose attitude is "What's the big deal about a baby? We have too many of them anyway. The whole thing now is just another biological process we can control at will."

With the current glamorization of sex, convenient forms of contraception, and the prevailing free-to-be philosophy of sexual relationships, the almost incredible complexities that lead to the birth of a child are too quickly forgotten. The reality is, of course, that there is nothing routine about conception and childbirth. The birth of a healthy child is dependent on a delicate balance of reproductive events that continues to awe the most sophisticated scientist. It is difficult to deny that there is at least a trace of miracle in the whole process. We simply cannot break down the reproductive process into cold biological facts.

Jane Lazarre in *The Mother Knot* offers an example of the continuing mystery human reproduction presents to medical scientists:

> My obstetrician had whispered a secret to me on a sunny afternoon. I had come to the office prepared with my written list of questions. . . . He answered wearily, "If you want answers to questions, have a miscarriage or toxemia or let something else go wrong with your pregnancy. We don't know anything about normal births." So much for technological know-how.

You will benefit from improving and expanding your knowledge about the male reproductive system, the production of sperm, the menstrual cycle, and events leading to conception and birth both in terms of the practical application it will have in sex selection and in terms of the deeper respect you will develop for yourself and your remarkable potential for creating new life.

XY = Male and Other Basics

The process of reproduction begins in the brain, with the *pituitary gland,* which sends hormonal messages to the male sex glands, or *testes.* These two glands develop inside a male baby's body before he is born and very gradually move downward, passing through a canal from the abdomen to the scrotum, which is outside the body. Occasionally this relocation is not complete by the time of birth, and surgery may be necessary to place the testes in their proper position so that sperm can be produced later in life. Additionally, in some instances the canal through which the testes pass does not close as tightly as it should—or, because of some type of strain, it is reopened. This condition (a special type of hernia) can usually be corrected by means of a simple surgical procedure.

Each of the testes is one to two inches long and shaped something like a plum, with a wide variation in size from man to man. The size of the glands, however, has nothing whatsoever to do with their ability to function. Similarly, one testicle may hang lower than the other, but this too is normal and is not a sign that the sex glands will have any difficulty performing their two functions, the secretion of male hormones and the production of sperm. (Likewise, physical construction has nothing whatever to do with the sex of offspring).

The *scrotum* is the pouch of loose skin that holds the testes. It may be "just skin," but it serves two important roles. First, this sac serves to hold and protect the delicate tissues of the testes. Second, it acts as a kind of thermostat, to make sure that the testes are always kept at about the same temperature, a few degrees *below* that of the rest of the body. The scrotum regulates the temperature both by means of its constantly functioning sweat glands and by acting as a sling that can raise or lower the glands as necessary. In bitter cold the muscular portion of the scrotum will automatically raise the testes, bringing them closer to the body. In warm surroundings the muscles will be more relaxed. And in *very* warm surroundings, if at all prolonged, there will be some destruction of sperm.

This intolerance to temperature extremes is, of course, the basis for the "hot shower" method of contraception, the idea being that the heat would immobilize the current sperm supply. But Mother Nature had too much foresight to risk the human race dying out from temporary applications of either heat or cold. As contraceptives, showers are only reliable when used in the manner of the old college joke about orange juice—not before, not after, but instead of.

SPERM PASSAGEWAYS

Once the sperm have been manufactured in the testes, they pass through five portions of a sperm passageway before they are released from the body: the epididymis, the vas deferens, the sperm "reservoir" or ampulla, the ejaculatory duct, and the urethra, which runs through the penis. In addition, two organs, the prostate gland and the seminal vesicles, donate liquid additives to the sperm.

The *epididymis,* which is really an extension of the tubes of the testes, is a twisted mass of coils which, if stretched out, would measure some sixteen to twenty feet. These coils provide the ideal surroundings for new sperm to grow and mature before they continue the journey that will end in their exit through the penis. When sperm first enter the epididymis they appear lifeless; yet in a matter of weeks, as a result of their exposure to the secretions of the walls of those tubes, they come to life somewhat. We must say "somewhat," because compared to what the sperm will be like later in their anatomical journey, when they leave the epididymis they are still relatively sleepy cells.

A Man's Reproductive Parts and the Organs near Them

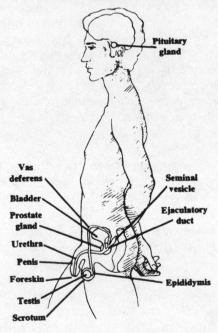

After about six weeks in the epididymis, the sperm enter the *vas deferens* and are moved by peristaltic contractions (a sort of rhythmic squeezing) up into the abdominal area, eventually entering the *ampulla.* Just prior to ejaculation, they are pushed into the *ejaculatory duct,* where they mix with secretions of the seminal vesicles and prostrate gland, and where they acquire their impressive ability to move by themselves. These secretions also prepare the sperm for the relatively hostile chemical environment of the female vagina. From the ejaculatory duct they are released through the *urethra* in the form of semen. The arrows in the diagram show you the rather circuitous route sperm take from the testes to the tip of the *penis.*

The Path of the Sperm

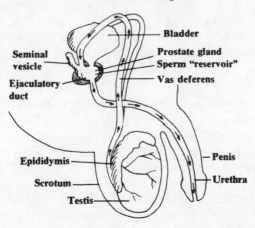

Bladder

Seminal vesicle

Prostate gland
Sperm "reservoir"

Ejaculatory duct

Vas deferens

Epididymis

Penis

Scrotum

Urethra

Testis

SPERMATOGENESIS

Since the sperm are the stars of the sex determination drama, it is worthwhile learning how they are formed and how they develop the ability to do what they do best.

Spermatogenesis, or sperm production, is set off by a hormone (interstitial-cell-stimulating hormone, or ICSH) sent by the pituitary via the bloodstream to the testes. Sperm do not suddenly come into existence when that hormone is released. The process is a gradual—and unique—one. Indeed, the development of a sperm cell is unlike that of any other cell in the body. In the course of their three-phase development, the male cells develop their potential for sex determination.

In *step one* the primitive cell (called a spermatogonium) divides to create identical cells. There is nothing unusual about this, because other cells in the body are constantly reproducing themselves. In this case, each of the new but still immature cells (known as primary spermatocytes) carries a full complement of cellular material, or chromosomes.

The chromosomes are the part of the cell where hereditary material (DNA) is kept. There are twenty-three pairs of chromosomes, making a total of forty-six. (Until 1956 the number of chromosomes in the human male and female was believed to be forty-eight instead of forty-six.) Only one of these pairs—two cells, one from each parent—is responsible for determining the child's sex if conception occurs.

During *step two,* under the influence of another pituitary hormone (follicle stimulating hormone, or FSH), the primary spermatocyte undergoes its unique process: it splits into two different cells, one carrying a

Y chromosome and the other an X. This secondary spermatocyte now has only *half* the number of chromosomes. These two "half cells" are identical, except that one carries the Y chromosome, the other the X chromosome. In *step three* these half cells split again, to form spermatids which eventually mature to become sperm.

If at the time of conception an X-bearing sperm fertilizes the egg, the child will be a girl. If a Y sperm fertilizes the egg, the child will be a boy. I emphasize that out of one spermatogonium, four spermatozoa are produced, two carrying the Y chromosome and two the X chromosome.* Thus there is *exactly* the same number of male- and female-producing sperm. Science offers no reason to suspect that for some genetic reason there might be more of one type or the other.

The sperm-making process is a continuous one (there is, however, some slowdown as a man gets older), but it takes a considerable amount of time—some seventy-four days—for primitive cells to complete this three-step process and become mature sperm.

In terms of interest in both fertility and sex selection, it is important to remember that during this long developmental process sperm are sensitive to conditions outside the man's body. For instance, excess heat is one threat. If tight jockey shorts push the testes and scrotum up next to the warmth of the body, the ideal temperature for sperm production is altered and the whole process is affected. This factor is particularly

---

*Medically, the X, or female-producing, sperm is known as a gynosperm; the Y, or male-producing sperm, as an androsperm. But for the sake of simplicity I will not be using those terms in this book.

Steps in Spermatogenesis

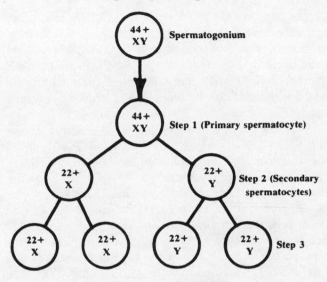

important for men whose fertility is marginal, who because of a low sperm count or some other factor may have difficulty fathering a child. The phenomenon has received regular attention in advice columns and elsewhere during the past few years, much to the gratitude of numerous couples who finally succeeded in conceiving after years of trying.

An interesting historical incident confirms the adverse effect that external stimuli can have on spermatogenesis.

In South America the Spanish conquerors who established the city of Potosi some 14,000 feet above sea level found to their dismay that they were unable to have children by the native women they married. Be-

cause local women married to local men were highly
fertile, it became apparent that it was the conquerors
who were sterile. Fifty-three years elapsed before children began to be born to women married to the Europeans. Apparently it took that long for their
physiological adjustment to the temperature change to
be completed. (The Spanish attributed the long-awaited
birth to a miracle performed by St. Nicholas of Tolen-
tino.)

As far as we know, X and Y sperm are affected
equally by temperature changes. Both types survive
best in conditions that are maintained naturally by the
contractions of the scrotum. There is no reason to
believe that a man with a lower than normal sperm
count, or semen which has been "depleted" by exces-
sive sexual activity, has a deficit of one or the other
type of sperm. You'll still hear stories to the contrary,
however—for instance, the frequently cited case of a
Persian ambassador with 100 wives at the court of St.
Petersburg, who produced 57 boys to 202 girls, a ratio
that could certainly have occurred by chance. (Almost
everyone knows at least one family that includes one
son and three or four daughters, or the reverse, a
corresponding ratio on a smaller scale.)

Similarly, both X and Y sperm appear to be about
equally influenced by all other environmental factors,
both before and after they are deposited in the vagina,
with one possible exception. It is well-known by fertility experts and other professionals that sperm are ad-
versely affected by the normally acid conditions of the
vagina. The survival of all sperm becomes limited at
varying rates, with *some* studies indicating that the
male Y sperm are particularly vulnerable. In the past
few years, however, reliable investigations have been

unable to confirm any difference, and the prevailing opinion among current experts is that X and Y have been created equal in this respect. The major holdout is Dr. Shettles, who still subscribes to his own axiom that baking soda douches produce boys and vinegar douches girls. In the absence of any proof, the generally accepted belief is that his (or any other) "successes" have been due to either a combination of other factors or to the simple phenomenon that even the woman who does nothing at all still retains a 50-50 chance of giving birth to the sex of her choice.

Researchers have studied such factors as initial sperm count, lifespan of the sperm after being deposited in the woman's body, age of the cervical secretions in the woman, and elasticity of cervical mucus, finding that none of these appears to discriminate between the X's and the Y's. (The changing texture of cervical mucus is important for a very different reason, however, as we will discuss in the next chapter.) The only significant behavioral difference uncovered to date has to do with motility. A handful of scientists still resist agreement, but the preponderance of evidence indicates that the Y's swim somewhat faster than the X's—a characteristic particularly useful in developing sex selection techniques, as well as artificial methods of sperm separation.

XX = Female (More Basics)

The female reproductive process also begins in the brain, with the small, bean-shaped pituitary gland. During childhood this gland is very active in releasing hormones which play a part in the regulation of almost every body function *except* those having to do with reproduction. Just before puberty, the pituitary gland "wakes up" and begins to send hormones through the bloodstream to the pelvic area to stimulate the ovaries, the female sex glands.

The female reproductive organs are arranged in the shape of a Y with curved arms. At the top of that super Y are the *ovaries,* two almond-shaped glandular organs an inch or so below the hipbone. The name "ovaries" (from the Latin word *ova,* meaning eggs) describes their function: the ovaries at the time of birth contain 200,000–400,000 egg cells and will release a few hun-

**A Woman's Reproductive Parts
and the Organs near Them**

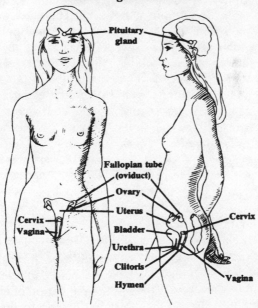

dred of them over the course of a woman's reproductive years.

Once the egg is released from the ovary, it enters one of the two *Fallopian tubes* or oviducts, each of which is four inches long and about as wide as a telephone cord. The Fallopian tubes are the "arms" in the Y configuration. These tubes, which are adjacent to the ovaries but not connected to them, have cilia (hairlike structures) that gently propel the egg toward the *uterus* or womb, an organ that is shaped like an upside-down pear. In a woman who has never had children, the uterus is about the size of a clenched fist; it is somewhat larger in a woman who has had children. The neck of the uterus, right at the point where the two arms of the Y meet, is the *cervix,* which connects with the *vagina,* a tubular organ usually about four inches long. The inner wall of the vagina is composed of highly elastic small folds or ridges which allow this organ to stretch during both sexual intercourse and childbirth. The vagina is kept moist by the tiny glands located deep within its inner walls, and by the secretions of *Bartholin's glands,* positioned very near the vagina, which contribute additional lubrication, particularly when a woman is sexually stimulated.

The vagina and the urethra (the passage through which urine is released) both open into an area called the *external genitalia,* the catchall name for a number of different structures. The *mons pubis,* a cushionlike mound of fat covered with pubic hair, is just above the *clitoris.* This tiny pea-shaped organ is made up of many nerve receptors and other sensitive tissue and has the capacity to become filled with blood and increase in size upon sexual arousal. The *labia majora* are two rounded folds of skin that extend from the mons pubis.

Inside the labia majora are the *labia minora,* which, along with the clitoris, respond during sexual excitement.

The Menstrual Cycle

We can best understand the events of the menstrual cycle by dividing it into three parts—Part 1 being the menstrual flow itself, Part 2 the events that take place before ovulation, and Part 3 all those events occurring after ovulation and just before the next menstrual period.

There is considerable confusion about the use of the terms cycle, period, and menstruation. The menstrual cycle is the time that elapses between the beginning of one menstrual bleeding episode and the beginning of the next. "Period" is the frequently used synonym for menstruation. I would prefer not to designate any particular cycle length here, because there is considerable variation, both from woman to woman and for the same woman at different times. For convenience, I sometimes use the twenty-eight-day cycle as our model, since this is the figure generally designated as "average." This in no way implies that cycles as short as three weeks or as long as seven weeks are considered abnormal, or even particularly unusual. It is important to remember, however, that in cycle lengths other than twenty-eight days the timing of menstrual events varies accordingly.

PART 1: THE MENSTRUAL PHASE
The most obvious part of the cycle is the menstrual phase, the five or so days of bleeding during which some two to three ounces of blood and other tissue are

released through the vagina. But other important events occur during those five days, too.

A couple of days after the flow begins, the pituitary gland releases the follicle stimulating hormone (FSH, the same hormone released by the male pituitary), which does exactly what its name implies: it causes the follicles or small sacs in the ovary to produce *estrogen,* which, among other things, signals the lining of the uterus, the *endometrium,* to start rebuilding itself.

The fact that the uterine lining can vary in consistency and appearance during the course of the menstrual cycle is related to the fact that it is supplied by two different types of blood vessels. One set serves the deepest portion of the uterus and is short and straight in appearance; these blood vessels function in a regular and continuous manner and do not take part in the rhythmic pattern of the menstrual cycle. The other vessels, which make up the outer portion of the endometrium, are larger and coiled in shape. Unlike the short, straight type, these blood vessels are highly susceptible to changes in the body's hormone levels.

PART 2: THE PROLIFERATIVE PHASE

Following the end of the menstrual flow, the levels of estrogen in the body increase even more significantly, and the large, coiled vessels in the endometrium respond. Indeed, their growth is so rapid at this time that the word "proliferate" is appropriate; thus the second part of the menstrual cycle is called the "proliferative phase."

While the uterine lining is rebuilding itself a number of the eggs in the follicles begin to grow. At first each of these selected eggs, surrounded by a thick protective

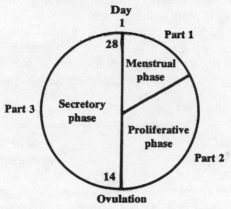

The Parts of a Menstrual Cycle

Day 1

Part 1

28

Menstrual phase

Part 3

Secretory phase

Proliferative phase

Part 2

14

Ovulation

membrane, is made up of one layer of cells, but as estrogen production continues the eggs get larger.

Near the end of this second phase of the cycle, about the thirteenth or fourteenth day of most, but not all, menstrual cycles, the pituitary responds to the high levels of estrogen by sending out the hormone LH or *luteinizing hormone*. The body has a sort of thermostat that controls the release of hormones. Just as a heater thermostat turns a heater on and off when the temperature in the room fluctuates, the female body's thermostat releases LH when a certain level of estrogen is attained.

LH appears to be responsible for choosing which of those growing eggs will be released each month (*usually* just one egg is chosen). And then LH works with FSH to bring about very rapid growth in that chosen egg. Within about twenty-four hours the egg is ripe and mature; it may look like a blister on the side of the ovary. At that point, approximately day fourteen or fifteen in a twenty-eight-day cycle, LH triggers *ovulation,* the release of the egg from the follicle.

The subject of ovulation—and the question of when it occurs—is critical to any attempt to influence the odds on your child's sex outcome; we will turn to it in detail in the next chapter.

PART 3: THE SECRETORY PHASE

Estrogen causes the glands in the uterine lining to secrete various chemicals. For this reason the third phase of the menstrual cycle is known as the *secretory phase*.

Once the egg leaves the ovary, the swaying cilia assist its descent down one of the two Fallopian tubes toward the uterus, a trip that will take some four to six days. It is here that sperm and egg will unite if they are to do so at all. Generally speaking, however, the egg only remains viable during the first twenty-four hours.

Following ovulation the pituitary hormone LH (which was responsible for triggering ovulation in the first place) transforms the follicle in which the egg grew into a bright orange-yellow structure called the *corpus luteum,* or "yellow body." Still under the influence of LH, the yellow body produces the second important female hormone, *progesterone,* which has a calming effect on the mild contractions normally experienced by the uterus.

Progesterone and estrogen team up to prepare the endometrium for arrival of the egg. By the time it reaches the uterus, the lining has built up considerably until it is soft, spongy, and engorged with blood. If conception occurred during the journey through the Fallopian tube the fertilized egg (now an *embryo*) has already begun to grow and can usually implant itself rather easily into the spongy uterine tissue. The increased blood supply is already waiting to nourish further growth and development.

If, however, the egg was not fertilized, LH is promptly withdrawn, estrogen and progesterone levels decline, the egg disintegrates, and the endometrial lining begins to deteriorate. This sloughing off of the unneeded blood-filled tissue produces the menstrual flow, which commences a short time later. Obviously, these seem like rather elaborate preparations to be so lightly discarded a large percentage of the time, but it is nature's way of ensuring optimal conditions for the embryo's survival as soon as they are needed. Note that the being who is eventually to become a baby is still referred to as an embryo during this early stage. Not until the end of the second month will the embryo become known as a *fetus.*

As you can tell from this discussion, the menstrual cycle follows a pattern of rising and falling hormone levels. With this shift in hormones many changes occur in the female body, but two in particular will be of interest to us in the next two chapters on the actual techniques for increasing the odds in sex preselection. These are: 1) the rise in body temperature which occurs once the levels of progesterone surge, and 2) changes in the quantity and consistency of the cervical mucus discharged from the vagina.

The following graphs give a summary of those hormonal changes in both a twenty-eight-day and a forty-day menstrual cycle. Note that the major variation in cycle length occurs *before* ovulation. In cycles of all lengths the number of days *after* ovulation is relatively constant, usually very close to fourteen.

Changes in the Levels of Estrogen and Progesterone During the Menstrual Cycle

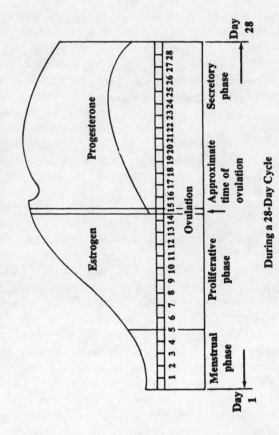

During a 28-Day Cycle

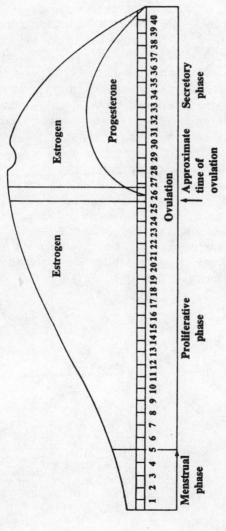

During a 40-Day Cycle

Those Two Reproductive Cells

When the egg leaves the ovary's follicle, it is well prepared to make the journey toward the uterus, having a food supply and a protective exterior to guard the vital chromosomal material in its nucleus. The egg cell is relatively large—about as large as the period at the end of this sentence. Compared to sperm and all other body cells, that's large. As we've already mentioned, the egg does not move under its own power; it depends on the Fallopian tubes' cilia for transport.

The sperm cell is different in many ways. First, there's not just one sperm present (as is usually the case with the egg). There are literally millions of them entering the female body as the result of just a single ejaculation. Some 66 to 867 million cells are present in the semen deposited during sexual intercourse.

Second, sperm cells are tiny—you'd need a high-powered microscope to see them. Third, they have the capacity to move on their own.

The Two Reproductive Cells

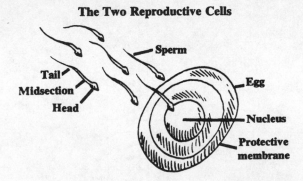

The sperm and the egg are different in another way too, a way that helps us answer the following major question.

WHEN CAN PREGNANCY OCCUR?

The egg has a relatively short lifetime. If it doesn't meet a sperm during the first twelve to twenty-four hours after ovulation, it disintegrates. During its first day of free floating, the egg doesn't get much beyond the first third of the Fallopian tube. And that's where the meeting of the egg and sperm usually takes place, if it happens at all.

Most medical texts state that sperm can survive about forty-eight hours once deposited in a woman's body. But recent research has led scientists to believe that *sperm may retain their capacity to fertilize an egg for ninety-six hours*—in some rare cases, possibly longer. This is a critical factor to keep in mind in your sex predetermination attempts. (It also explains some of those pregnancies that "couldn't have happened.") So in making our estimates here of the fertile period—and thus answering the question about when conception can occur—let's use the most probable survival periods: twenty-four hours for the ovum, ninety-six hours for the sperm. To estimate the possible pregnancy period we add these two intervals:

96 hours	+ 24 hours	= 120 hours (5 days)
estimated maximum fertilization capacity of the sperm	approximate survival period of the egg	in each menstrual cycle when sexual intercourse could lead to pregnancy

The first twenty-four-hour period is the one immediately following ovulation. The other ninety-six hours are those occurring *before* the egg is released. In other words, even though the sperm may be early arrivals, they patiently wait for the egg to appear—and some of them are able to linger for as long as four days. For the fertile period to extend through the fifth day, however, the troops must be replenished in the interim.

If you are puzzled about why we added the intervals to estimate the full length of the fertile period, perhaps this illustration will help.

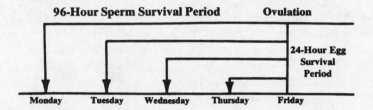

If you have sexual intercourse without a contraceptive on Monday and ovulate the following Friday, it is possible that some of Monday's sperm will be alive and well, waiting in the Fallopian tubes when the egg is released. Intercourse on Tuesday, Wednesday, or Thursday increases the probability that sperm will be present at the right (or wrong, depending on your point of view) time.

We should note here in talking about a ninety-six-hour fertile period that all those hours *do not have* an equal probability of conception. Certainly intercourse on Thursday or Friday would carry a much greater likelihood of conception than intercourse earlier in the week.

No matter how long the menstrual cycle, whether it is twenty-four or forty days, there are still only five days when sexual intercourse can lead to pregnancy. And, of course, a single act of intercourse cannot encompass the full five days. Sperm introduced at any other time of the month will encounter only failure for one of two reasons: Either there is no egg available, or by the time there is, the sperm have deteriorated to a point where they are too feeble to fertilize anything.

BOY? OR GIRL? THE SPERM DECIDE

I've presented this outline of reproductive physiology in preparation for the discussion here and in the next chapter of the biological factors that determine whether a child will be male or female.

Sperm play the key role in the sex predetermination drama, although that information has not been common knowledge for long.

In 1676 sperm cells were first identified by a medical student named Ham, who examined a sample of human semen under Anthony van Leeuwenhoek's simple microscope. Once the tiny cells were found, Leeuwenhoek reported his observations to the Secretary of the Royal Society of London. Being sensitive to the morality of his time, he was discreet in his announcement: "What I have here described was not obtained by a sinful contrivance on my part, but the observations were made upon the excess with which Nature provided me in my conjugal relations. And if your Lordship should consider such matters either disgusting or likely to seem offensive to the learned, I earnestly beg they be regarded as private and either published or suppressed, as your Lordship's judgment dictates."

Leeuwenhoek's material was published, but research on the role of sperm was confused by the prevailing controversy over whether sperm were related to fertility, or whether each sperm cell itself contained a complete miniature human being that just needed to be "planted" in the female womb so that it could grow. After Leeuwenhoek found sperm in human semen, observers claimed they could see miniature dogs, cats, horses, or whatever in the semen of other species. (So much for the power of suggestion!)

It was not until almost a hundred years later that an Italian biologist, Lazarro Spallanzani, performed what should have been a crucial experiment: he made tiny pairs of "trousers" out of a waxed fabric and put them on male frogs before he mated them with females. The eggs were not fertilized, but when Spallanzani collected the semen that had been deposited in the frog trousers, he found he could fertilize the frog eggs with it by laboratory procedures. Spallanzani showed that physical contact with semen was necessary for reproduction, but there was still the question of whether it was the sperm cell or some other portion of the seminal fluid that was critical for fertilization. Not until 1923 was it determined that sperm are of two different varieties and that it is whether they carry an X or a Y sex chromosome that determines the sex of the new child.

But even in the 1980s much remains to be discovered, particularly in the area of sperm motility. In laboratory conditions sperm swim relatively slowly. If they were to move at the same rate of speed under the actual conditions of intercourse, it would take them several hours to reach the Fallopian tubes, even assuming that they continually move in the correct direction (which they sometimes do not). This observation is in direct contrast with the well-known fact that within just a few *minutes* after sexual intercourse, sperm can be found in the Fallopian tubes. (The *average* time is sixty to ninety minutes.) The question, then, is how they get there so fast. It seems obvious that they do not move completely on their own. It has been suggested that a chemical in semen, *prostaglandin,* plays an important role in sperm transport by stimulating the uterus in such a way that sperm are sucked in through the cervix and up to the Fallopian tubes.

We need to know more about how sperm get from the vagina to the ovum where they have the opportunity to fertilize. Once we have more answers in this area, we'll have clues as to why, in varying circumstances, either X or Y sperm might have some special advantage during their uphill travels.

THE TRAVELS OF THE SPERM

As I've pointed out, in the course of ejaculation millions of sperm enter a woman's body. It may seem that nature was overgenerous in deciding on the number of sperm, given that only one is necessary to fertilize an egg, but this large number is needed for two reasons.

First, as the sperm in their alkaline environment reach the acidic conditions of the vagina, they generally encounter a very hostile reception. Although the chemicals in semen neutralize much of the acid in the vaginal secretions, a number of sperm die right then and there. The reduced number of sperm (though still in the thousands) that go on to enter the more alkaline uterus is further diminished because half of them enter the "wrong" Fallopian tube, the one that isn't transporting the egg that month. Of the 66 to 867 million sperm deposited during intercourse, fewer than a hundred are present in the tube at the time the egg and sperm join forces—a reduction of about 99.9 percent. This clearly illustrates why men with low sperm counts often experience fertility problems.

Second, a large number of sperm are needed because, although only one enters the egg, the efforts of a number of them are necessary to break down the protective wall of the egg and allow fertilization to occur.

A Closer Look at the X and Y Sperm

As I emphasized earlier, there are two types of sperm, one class with an X chromosome, the other with a Y. A Y-bearing sperm unites with the egg to form a boy; an X-bearing sperm unites with the egg to form a girl. At the moment of conception, while he or she is still a single cell, one of the most important factors in a person's life is determined. And it is clear that *this important characteristic is determined by the father,* not the mother, a fact which, had it been known a few hundred years ago, might have saved the heads of Anne Boleyn and other daughter-producing queens.

Referring back to the discussion of spermatogenesis, you already know that every spermatocyte produces exactly 50 percent X's and 50 percent Y's. They meet with the XX egg in the fashion shown in the diagram opposite.

The result: 50 percent XX; 50 percent XY. And there is no way around it, no "hidden" factors that under normal conditions can reduce the production of either X- or Y-type sperm.

It is only very recently that we have had access to a technique for accurately identifying the X and Y

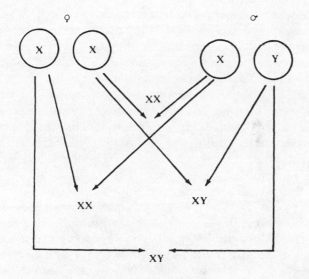

♀ ♂

XX

XX   XY

XY

sperm. In the 1960s, Dr. Landrum B. Shettles thought he had uncovered a simple method for distinguishing between the two types by using a phase contrast microscope. According to his highly publicized contention, those sperm with small round heads contained Y chromosomes, those with large oval heads carried X chromosomes. But like a great many other oversimplified theories, this one was perched on shaky legs. Continuing research by the world's leading authorities failed to validate Shettles's report, and with today's sophisticated equipment it can now be clearly refuted.

Commenting on the subject in a 1971 issue of *Fertility and Sterility,* a Yale Medical School team noted that a number of scientists had concluded that "Shettles was observing a phase contrast optical aberration," not a distinction between X and Y sperm. Other researchers have noted that sperm (of either "sex") are not uniform in size, and that a certain amount of variation in both weight and volume can be created by varying metabolic products within the cell membrane. In *Getting Pregnant in the 1980s,* Drs. Robert H. Glass and Ronald J. Ericsson acknowledge that the X chromosome itself is somewhat larger than the Y chromosome, but that this difference is "infinitesimal compared to the overall weight of the sperm." The considerable variation in size among *all* sperm is far greater than could be accounted for by the differences in the chromosome (i.e., sex) portions alone.

But progress marches on. In 1970, two British researchers, Dr. Peter Barlow of Guy's Hospital Medical School, and Dr. C. G. Vosa of the Botany School at Oxford University, succeeded in developing a chemical test to identify the two types of sperm. Human semen supplied by volunteers was stained with a substance called quinacrine mustard. Microscopic analysis under a mercury vapor or ultraviolet light revealed a fluorescent spot in the heads of about half the sperm which was much brighter than the fluorescent material in the rest of the sperm head. This spot they named the F-body and later demonstrated that it indicates the presence of the male-producing chromosome. (More recently, a few researchers have been investigating a similar "spot," known as the B-body.)

The photograph on the following page (supplied through the courtesy of Drs. Barlow and Vosa) shows what a stained semen specimen looks like under the microscope. The sperm heads you can see "glowing" are Y, or male-producing, sperm.

No parallel staining technique has yet been developed for identification of female-producing sperm except, of course, that they can be distinguished by the absence of the F-body. This negative method—based

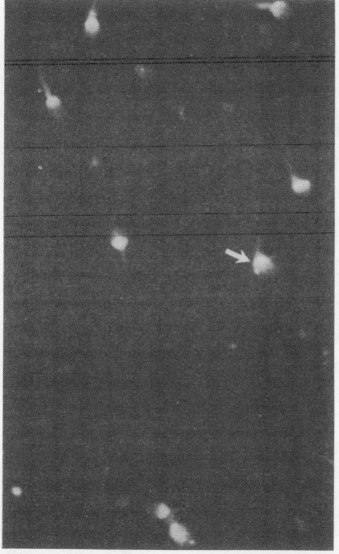

Photo supplied courtesy of Dr. Peter Barlow and Dr. C. G. Vosa.
When human semen is stained, the Y sperm take on a fluorescent look.

on what is not there—is not really an intended slight by chauvinistic male researchers; it just turned out that way. But it does have some interesting anthropological connotations: of the many species of animal semen examined, only two besides man exhibit the F-body characteristic—the gorilla and a type of field mouse known as a vole.

Events of the 20th century have unlocked many doors that lead us ever closer to solving the riddle of human sex selection. In the male, we have greatly increased our overall knowledge of spermatogenesis, including the role of sperm in sex determination; in the female, we have a much clearer understanding of the importance of ovulation and timing within the menstrual cycle. We're still a long way from all the answers about the X vs. Y race, but until a full explanation is available, the facts that we *do* have can be used to advantage. The science of reproductive physiology has revealed some specific and practical techniques that can increase the chances of having either a boy baby or a girl baby. That's what the next two chapters are all about.

4

Beating Those 50-50 Odds: The Basics

Sex determination advice of the past often focused, as we have noted, on nutritional regimens, the adjusting of relative "parental strength," autosuggestion, and coital positions that would challenge a professional acrobat. Two equally ancient techniques, variations of which have survived through the ages, are being given serious consideration today as important variables in determining the sex of the forthcoming child: first, *the timing of sexual intercourse within the menstrual cycle,* and second, *changes within the woman's vagina* before and during intercourse.

The recommendations here stem from these two factors. Both the information and advice, however, are based on a series of recent international studies and are quite different from earlier suggestions about the association between timing of intercourse and the sex of the baby.

Before we get to the specifics of "how to," let's consider first some of the scientific background on the questions of chemical changes and the timing of intercourse, and then the nature of the evidence that has advanced our knowledge to where it is today. It is worth taking the time for this, because you are bound to hear conflicting advice—either from friends and relatives who specialize in old wives' tales, or from those who have been reading sex determination guides that have now been outdated by new medical research.

A Chemical Reaction: Some Earlier Thoughts

Two pieces of advice about the effect of chemistry on sex outcome have been offered for the past few decades, although the roots go back much farther. First, altering the chemical balance (the pH) of the female reproductive tract through douching with either a solution of baking soda for a boy or white vinegar for a girl was presumed to be a critical step in sex control. Second, early and frequent female orgasm supposedly favors male births.

ON ACIDITY AND ALKALINITY

The chemical symbol pH is used for the scale, ranging from 0 to 14, that measures a substance's alkalinity or acidity. A substance with a pH of 7 is neutral; anything less than 7 is increasingly acid; greater than 7, increasingly alkaline. For instance, the pH of lemon juice is about 2.3, vinegar 2.9, pure water 7.0; a baking soda and water mixture may have a pH of 8 or 9 or more.

In the early 1930s Dr. Felix Unterberger, a German obstetrician and professor at Mercy Hospital in Königsberg, noticed that a number of women who were having difficulty becoming pregnant had unusually acid vaginal secretions and wondered if this could be incapacitating the sperm before they had a chance to travel through the cervix. He advised these women to use alkaline douches before sexual intercourse, and in many cases the women became pregnant. But what was even more interesting than the increase in fertility was Dr. Unterberger's report that almost all the patients who conceived after following his douching advice delivered boys. Specifically, over a ten-year period fifty-three out of fifty-four patients who did conceive had male babies. (It was reported that the one girl was born to a woman who was pregnant before she applied the douching advice.) Soon after the publication of Unterberger's findings a Bavarian obstetrician "confirmed" the effect of precoital douching, and two British gynecologists published an article in *Lancet* indicating that there might indeed be something to the Unterberger hypothesis; maybe alkaline solutions *did* favor male conceptions.

The research was highly publicized in 1932, when a doctor from Rotterdam, while attending the Sixth International Genetics Conference in Ithaca, New York, gave an impromptu lecture on the subject on the steps of a Cornell University building. The press immediately took note, and in the days that followed, the "baking-soda-boy" theory got more attention than all the formal conference papers combined. The American Genetic Association and other professional groups reported a "Christmas-like flurry of mail asking if this advice was scientifically accurate." Everyone was excited about what appeared at the time to be a real breakthrough in the quest for sex control. The fervor even entered the world of international affairs; when Emperor Hirohito of Japan, who had apparently established friendly contacts with the Sun God, was rewarded with a male heir, birth control advocate Margaret Sanger claimed joint credit with the Sun God because she had written a letter to his majesty explaining the virtues of soda bicarb.

The baking soda-vinegar method received another boost in 1937, when the president of the *New York Daily News* became personally interested in the subject. He consulted several geneticists and concluded that there was enough to the theory to warrant his commissioning the Applied Laboratories in Dayton, New York, to do the necessary experiments to find out whether precoital douching was the answer.

The first experiments began in 1938, and the results were presented almost on a day-by-day basis by one Carl Warren, who became known as the *News*'s "Sex Control Editor." But alas, the results were conflicting, and despite the publication of two books that enthusiastically supported the method (Warren wrote his own book, *Animal Sex Control,* and D. H. Sandell, M.D., contributed his *Boy or Girl: How Parents Can Decide the Sex of Their Child* to the growing library of how-to sex determination books), the theory succumbed to the criticism of an increasing number of scientists. For instance, the editor of the *Journal of Heredity* went on record as saying he would eat a full issue of his admittedly dry journal if the animal experiments (which he termed "veritable laboratory blitzkrieg") ever confirmed the Unterberger theory.

Since Dr. Unterberger's report in the 1930s there has

been little evidence supporting the idea that douching can influence the sex of one's offspring. Indeed, research over the last five years by several of the world's foremost reproduction specialists suggests that we may have been on the wrong track entirely in this regard. Nevertheless, the *theory* is very much alive and continues to receive regular attention in the popular media. As I mentioned in Chapter 3, the chief proponent is Dr. Shettles, but he is becoming hard put to find professional supporters who fully agree with him today.

If you were to conduct your own survey, it would take you no time at all to find a woman who has herself produced a "baking-soda-boy," or knows someone who has. Most of these people are unaware that their "success" was probably less likely due to what was in the douche as to *when* the douche was used. Baking soda can help to increase the probability of conception because it creates in the vagina an environment more compatible with that to which the sperm has been accustomed. But, according to our best evidence right now, this holds true for *both* X and Y types. The alleged success rate is about as startling as a race between two turtles: it may take a while, but it's a pretty safe bet that eventually one or the other of them is going to win. Hypothetically, there does remain the possibility that pH might affect some other factor that in turn could favor either the X or Y sperm. However, that suggestion is nothing more than conjecture at this point.

ON FEMALE ORGASM AND SEX OUTCOME

The Talmud, completed between the fourth and sixth centuries A.D., may have been the first source to recommend that early female orgasm favors male births. It states that "the determination of sex takes place at the moment of cohabitation. When the woman emits her semen before the man, the child will be a boy. Otherwise it will be a girl." What exactly underlies this theory is a matter of speculation. Perhaps it was thought that the female secretions somehow led to the conception of a son, or possibly there was a bit of the "superior opposites" philosophy mixed in—the notion that if the woman achieved orgasm first she would engender a child of the opposite sex.

The theory of female-orgasm-first remained intermittently popular. In 1885 Samuel Hough Terry's book, *Controlling Sex in Generation: The Physical Law Influencing the Embryo of Man and Brute and Its Direction to Produce Male or Female Offspring at Will,* explained that when women got "charged up" they inevitably had a boy, or, as one of Terry's associates so aptly summarized it, "I know when my wife is conceiving a boy because she does all the work." He too refers to that story of the woman who was being sued for divorce because of an illegitimate child and her lawyer's explanation that the young man had grasped her by the hand and "straightaway such a thrill went through her whole body that she had no control over herself." This circumstance, Terry notes confidently, was the ideal one for a male birth. Indeed, if a woman had only daughters Mr. Terry expressed his sympathy, because she was obviously inexperienced in the "electrical" thrills of female climax.

In 1886 the *Edinburgh Medical Journal* published an anecdotal report of a warlike tribe which had had a particularly successful raid, killing all of the males in the enemy's camp. The victors then married the widows of the slain men and subsequently had children by

them. The sex ratio of these offspring was highly unusual: 403 females to 79 males. Perhaps, suggested the
authors, this was due to the fact that the captive wives
were in no frame of mind to experience orgasm during
sexual relations.

In 1911 P. J. McElrath's book, *The Key to Sex Control,* caused renewed interest in the relationship of sex
outcome to female orgasm, although his basic theory
was so complex that probably not too many users
understood his premise.

McElrath wrote that fresh sperm were by definition
male producing, and as they aged and got weaker they
(naturally) became female sperm: "When females fail
to reach orgasm, the old, thick mucous secretions remain in the uterine cavity and render it difficult for the
sperm to make their way into the Fallopian tubes . . .
the delay consumes the nutrition stored in the nuclei of
the sperm, the heads are reduced in size and consequently they are rendered female-producing." Thus
female orgasm served the purpose of clearing the chan-
nels so the fresh, young, vibrant male sperm could race
to their goal before the inevitable female deterioration
set in.

McElrath had both "evidence" to back up his theory
and some advice on how to implement it. He reported
that Jews had more boys, and claimed that this was no
surprise to him because Jewish men are circumcised;
the tip of the penis is left bare and becomes less sensitive, and therefore ejaculation is slower, allowing
women to have an orgasm first. On the other hand,
prostitutes had more than the expected number of girls
because "a male does not seek a harlot until the ves-
iculae seminales are distended with aged spermatozoa."

McElrath's followers were advised to take "an alcoholic stimulant" to help in the proper orgasm orchestration: if a boy was desired, the woman should have a few stiff drinks before bedtime to reduce her chances of orgasm; if a daughter was planned, it was the husband who should drink heartily from the fruits of the vine.

In 1953, August J. von Borosini revived the orgasm theory and speculated that women with many husbands had more boys because they obviously had more sex, which would increase their odds on orgasm. He thought the old French proverb which says that boys are conceived before midnight, girls after, made good biological sense because after midnight women were too tired to achieve full sexual satisfaction. But as so often happens in the area of sex selection, von Borosini had an opinion but no facts to back him up.

The question for us is as follows: What do we now know about the relationship of female climax and sex outcome? Do female sexual secretions, particularly at orgasm, make the vagina more alkaline and thus, in theory, more friendly to male-producing sperm?

The only thing we are really sure of is that the results of some inquiries in this area have been conflicting. For instance, studies of artificial insemination show a higher than expected proportion of male births; interestingly, the proportion of males was once reported to be as high as 160 to 100 when the husband's sperm was used and only 140 to 100 when an anonymous donor's sperm was selected. Some researchers suggest that the use of the husband's sperm "puts women in a happy frame of mind," creating a chemical condition akin to orgasm, and that this "manifests itself genitally by the secretion of more cervical fluid, hence a more alkaline medium."

The theory relating to orgasm sounds great, but unfortunately it has not yet survived the rigors of experimental testing, primarily because *we have no evidence that female orgasm causes any chemical change whatever in the vagina.* One group of researchers (who obviously had some very cooperative subjects) inserted devices inside women's vaginas just prior to intercourse, so that they could monitor any chemical changes that took place. They found that when the woman's sex partner used a condom and she experienced orgasm, there was absolutely no change in acidity or alkalinity in the vagina. When there was intercourse without contraception, the pH changed dramatically, but not as a result of orgasm. It was the introduction of semen into the vagina that changed the pH from slightly acid (4.3) to just about neutral (7.2).

Moreover, scientists have failed to establish any other type of chemical change created by orgasm, nor have they been able to discover any physical change that might possibly favor one type of sperm over the other. This is not to say that none exists, only that if there are any discriminating factors, we don't know about them yet.

Coital Timing and Sex Outcome

What of the advice about timing, various versions of which have survived through the ages?

Now that we've covered some of the factors that *aren't* relevant (as far as we know), we now arrive at one that definitely *is*. Like many attempts at sex selection, however, the insemination timing theories have a number of contradictory variations. All this contradiction and confusion is understandable, however, if you bear in mind that until 1930 the processes of ovulation and menstruation were generally assumed to be a single event, or at least that they occurred at the same time.

SOME EARLIER IDEAS

Hippocrates was possibly the first to argue that male births were more likely to result from coitus in the days immediately after the end of the menstrual flow. As one medical history puts it:

> Hippocrates writes in his booke (concerning superfoetation) of the means how to get a man or woman child. Hee that will beget a son must know his wife as soon as her courses were staved, and then try to the utmost of his strength; but if hee desire to get a daughter, hee must company with his wife a good while after her courses or at the time when she hath them.

During the early part of this century there was a flutter of excitement about some observations which seemed to suggest that Hippocrates had the right idea. The War Office supplied a group of German researchers with the dates on which the husbands in their study series were home on leave. Assuming that the couples had intercourse when the husband was at home, the researchers calculated "insemination dates" and reported, in a number of different studies, that conceptions occurring in the first ten days of the menstrual cycle yielded up to 84 percent male births. (See the table later in this chapter for a summary of some of these studies. You'll also note that a similar study was done much earlier, in 1878.)

But while these data were being presented and evaluated, the contemporary authors whom I mentioned in Chapter 1 were, with very little if any empirical evidence, insisting that mid-cycle insemination yielded male births. For instance, Louis Dechmann (who took out a copyright on his formula) thought that the sex would be opposite of that of the weaker cell. He hypothesized that "since an egg released during the menstrual flow" (!) would deteriorate over the course of the next two weeks, intercourse at mid-cycle would lead to the fertilization of a tired old egg. This tired egg would then "lose" the struggle and lead to conception of a child of the opposite sex, in this case a male.

And to complete the gamut of possibilities, there were those who recommended that sex a week or so *before* the menstrual period would yield males. McElrath's *The Key to Sex Control* advised this approach. Again, he thought menstruation and ovulation were basically the same event. If you had sex just before the flow, he reasoned, you might have a chance of triggering ovulation well before it would have occurred spontaneously, "during the five days of bleeding," and thus you'd increase your chances of fertilizing a nice, fresh, newly released egg, which of course would produce a boy! Speaking sociologically, McElrath said that conceptions occurring during the first month of marriage were more likely to be male because it was the prevailing custom to schedule weddings about two weeks after the menstrual flow ended. Conversely, illegitimate births were more likely to be female, because harlots were less likely to abstain from sex in the days during and just after the flow, thus increasing the probability of fertilizing a "stale" (female-producing) egg.

BEWARE OF METHODS THAT DON'T WORK!

During the 1950s and 1960s the late Dr. Sophia Kleegman of New York University Medical School did considerable research in the area of human artificial insemination. Part of her technique (as in all artificial insemination attempts) was to perform the insemination procedure as close as possible to the time of ovulation. She determined ovulation using basal body temperature readings (in the same way I'll describe later in this chapter), but she did not use changes in cervical mucus discharge as additional evidence. (We will also be using this method of ovulation detection.) Her patients demonstrated an interesting and unexpected trend: up to 80 percent of those who conceived as a result of insemination on the day of ovulation or the day before ovulation delivered male babies.* A Japanese gynecologist named Yoshida has confirmed Kleegman's findings of more males when artificial insemination was used around the time of ovulation.

As I mentioned in the introduction, as a result of his own laboratory attempts to identify male- and female-producing sperm, and calling on Dr. Kleegman's results with artificial insemination, Dr. Shettles (with medical writer David Rorvik) set forth his advice on how to have a male baby. His book, *Your Baby's Sex: Now You Can Choose,* and the more recent update, *Choose Your Baby's Sex,* indicated that insemination immediately before ovulation favored male births, whereas earlier insemination more frequently resulted in female babies.

---

*The observation that artificial insemination yields more male births was not a new one. An article in a 1941 issue of the *Journal of the American Medical Association* reported that the ratio of males to females was 8:5 with this method.

Shettles and Rorvik stated that:

> . . . with exposure to pregnancy two to twenty-four hours before ovulation, the babies were predominantly male (78 percent); with exposure to pregnancy thirty-six or more hours before ovulation, the babies were predominantly female.

Their advice, then, was that couples wanting a boy engage in coitus just before the moment of ovulation, when the egg is high in the Fallopian tube, and that those wanting a daughter do so in the early part of the cycle, avoiding the day or days just prior to ovulation.

These recommendations were interesting, and in the absence of other more established advice, couples eagerly tried the "Shettles method."

For example, one respected gynecologist in Texas began advising his patients to follow the procedure for having boys. When I talked with him he was so upset over the results that he had given up recommending it. The first thirty couples who had followed the Shettles advice and had sexual intercourse as close to ovulation as possible had had girls! One of his patients, an artist, had taken the formula so seriously that she put it into graphic form showing how Y spermatozoa were leapfrogging the X ones.

From the time this method was first introduced to the public, scientists had several reservations about it. First, the advice contradicted both those early German studies and all animal studies, which showed that it was *early,* not late, insemination that favored a male birth. Second, Rorvik and Shettles had generally relied on Dr. Kleegman's cases, which were based almost exclusively on artificial insemination. In the majority of cases Dr. Shettles had not tested his methods on couples who conceived as a result of sexual intercourse.

Third, and potentially more serious, concentrating intercourse relatively late in the cycle—that is, on the day of or the day after ovulation—may carry with it some undesirable side effects. There is reason to believe that an egg begins to deteriorate soon after it is released from the ovary. If a couple is avoiding intercourse until they feel ovulation has already occurred, they may be increasing the possibility of fertilizing an old, over-ripe egg and assuming an increased risk of miscarriage and other problems.

At the end of the twenty-four hours following ovulation, the egg—if it is still viable at all—has undergone probable chromosomal and other pathological changes that dramatically increase the odds of birth defects and other disorders if conception should occur. This phenomenon has been suggested as a cause of at least some cases of Downs syndrome (which is itself the result of a chromosome abnormality). Much more research needs to be done in this area, and much is in progress, but we already understand enough to know that it is a good idea to avoid sexual intercourse on the day or two immediately following ovulation or, if you prefer, to use a mechanical form of contraception.

Human Sex Selection: Our Latest Information

THE TIMING OF INTERCOURSE AND YOUR BABY'S SEX

During the late 1960s Dr. Rodrigo Guerrero V. began to collect information on the sex outcome of conceptions taking place during various portions of the menstrual cycle. Specifically, he collected statistics on two groups of women: first, those who had been artificially inseminated, generally because of a fertility problem, and second, those who were having normal sexual intercourse, following the "temperature-rhythm" method to detect ovulation.

By temperature, I am referring to the woman's basal body temperature, or BBT, which is the thermometer reading immediately upon waking in the morning. Women practicing natural family planning methods routinely collect this information, as do artificial insemination patients. The readings are charted on a graph and the resultant curve used to predict ovulation. A sudden temperature shift indicates that ovulation has occurred. The technique is of little use, however, unless specific instructions are followed, which will be explained a little later.

Two specific types of information were critical: (1) the date the insemination occurred (whether done artificially in a physician's office or in sexual intercourse) in relation to the woman's basal body temperature curve, and (2) the sex of the baby conceived.

Initially the results were puzzling: when the records of artificially and naturally inseminated women were analyzed together, there appeared to be no relationship whatever between the time of insemination and sex outcome; that is, there seemed to be no particular "boy" or "girl" days. But when artificially and naturally inseminated women were considered *separately,* the results were startling. There was indeed a significant shift in probabilities of boy and girl births by insemination timing, but unexpectedly, the results with natural and artificial insemination were the opposite.

With natural insemination the probability of a male

birth rose to *over 68 percent* when the "responsible" sexual intercourse took place five or more days before ovulation. When coitus took place the day of ovulation, only 43.5 percent of the babies were boys; in other words, the percentage of girls increased to 56 or 57 percent. On the other hand, among infants conceived from artificial insemination at or about the time of ovulation, boys predominated (62 percent). These results withstood rigid statistical analysis and were confirmed by subsequent studies; they are extremely unlikely to be chance observations.

When early studies that appeared to contradict these findings were reanalyzed using the same methods, all conflicts were resolved. It is apparent now that the earlier confusion about the timing for "boy" and "girl" days in relation to ovulation was due to the fact that different researchers were using different definitions of when ovulation was occurring and how long the possible fertile period was. No attention was given to the *type* of insemination used, whether artificial or natural.

For instance, Dr. Franciszek Benendo, writing in *Polish Endocrinology* in 1970, identified the time of ovulation as "fourteen days before the beginning of the menstrual flow" and concluded that inseminations at the time of ovulation increased the odds on a male birth. This conclusion was initially interpreted as being contradictory to the Guerrero conclusions and supportive of the Shettles method. A closer look, however, revealed that his methodology was different from both Guerrero's and Dr. Shettles's. All women *do not* ovulate "fourteen days before the beginning of the menstrual flow." The only practical and relatively dependable way of determining ovulation is with a basal body temperature curve.

There is at least one other example of how different

definitions of when ovulation occurs can affect the results of a sex predetermination study. Dr. Melvin R. Cohen intensively studied the sex outcome of babies born as a result of artificial insemination, but could find no surge in male births "around the time of ovulation." But when Dr. Guerrero reanalyzed Dr. Cohen's data using the temperature shift as the indicator of when ovulation occurred, the "inconsistency" disappeared.

NATURAL INSEMINATION VS. ARTIFICIAL INSEMINATION

The following graph, "Percent of Males at Birth," uses zero as the day of temperature shift. As you can

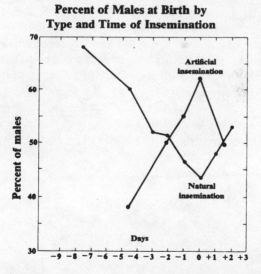

Percent of Males at Birth by Type and Time of Insemination

"Day 0" here is the day of the upward shift in basal body temperature. As you can see, the patterns for artificial and natural insemination are reversed.

see, the two kinds of insemination resulted in very
different sex ratios. With artificial insemination the
percentage of male offspring was highest on the day of
the shift in basal body temperature, that is, the day
after the probable time of ovulation. On that same day,
the percentage of male children conceived in sexual
intercourse was at its lowest point.

Studies that have used the actual day of ovulation as
the "zero" point do not, of course, illustrate this phenomenon so clearly. (The figures would be comparable
to those given for the " −1" day on the graph.) Instead
they tend to muddle the overall picture because the
results of the two techniques are contradicting each
other.

Two trends are immediately obvious in these percentages. First, the closer you get to the shift in temperature, the lower the odds on the conception of a
male child with natural insemination. Second, at no
point do the probabilities of a female birth go higher
than 56 or 57 percent.

The variation in percentages of male and female
births relative to the shift in temperature in cases of
natural insemination was as follows:

**Probable time
of ovulation**

Number of days before the shift in temperature

	−9	−8	−7	−6	−5	−4	−3	−2	−1	0	+1
Percentage of male births	←———68.3———→				←—60.5—→		52	51.3	48	43.5	48
Percentage of female births	←———31.7———→				←—39.5—→		48	48.7	52	56.5	52

It should be noted that the total number of births resulting from intercourse more than five days before ovulation is going to be relatively low. Why nature tends to favor male births under these circumstances is still unknown, but we can assume that for some reason more than twice as many Y's and X's are apparently able to remain viable during the "waiting period" for the egg's arrival.

The key to implementing advice on the "right" timing of coitus lies in predicting the days when boys or girls are more likely to be conceived. Before you can do that you must have an answer to the basic question: When does ovulation occur?

Predicting Ovulation

Ovulation prediction is often difficult but for nearly all women it is not impossible. Generally, the most reliable methods are the basal body temperature and changes in cervical secretions, but for some there are other aids in meeting the challenge.

THROUGH MITTELSCHMERZ

Some women have a sharp pain in their abdomen (known by the German word *Mittelschmerz,* pain in the mid-cycle), which may indicate that ovulation is in process. The pain, when it does occur, presumably represents the rupture of the egg from the follicle, just before it enters the Fallopian tube.

Only some 15 percent of the female population experiences *Mittelschmerz,* so for most this method is highly unreliable. If your period is very regular and you are anticipating the "signal," you might notice it. But if it occurs at all, it can easily be confused with a fleeting cramp or slight touch of indigestion.

WITH A CALENDAR

With the second method, it is possible to get a *general idea* of when ovulation will take place by simply counting calendar days. Most women ovulate *fourteen or fifteen days before the beginning of the next menstrual cycle*. Technically, it is more accurate to say that ovulation occurs somewhere between twelve and sixteen days before the last day of the menstrual cycle, that is, the day before the beginning of the next menstrual flow. But fourteen days falls in the middle and is usually applied as an average for identifying ovulation.

If, for instance, your last menstrual period began on November 27, you might estimate that you ovulated about November 12 or 13. Of course that is backwards information, like asking someone on a bus which stop Main Street is and being told to watch him and get off two stops before he does. But there is a way to use this backwards information in conjunction with some other clues.

Fortunately, nature tends to be regular, so you can hope that the same information will apply to the next cycle as well. If a woman's period begins November 27 and she has a regular twenty-eight-day cycle, she'll expect her period again on December 25. She might predict that she will ovulate about two weeks before that, or on December 10 or 11.

On the other hand, if the cycles are thirty-two or thirty-three days long, we can substract fourteen and estimate that ovulation will occur around day 18 or 19. Ovulation does not really occur "in the middle of the cycle," as is so often said. The general rule is "fourteen or fifteen days before the beginning of the next men-

Predicting Ovulation in a 28-Day Cycle

NOVEMBER

	1*	2*	3*	4*	5*	6
7	8	9	10	11	12	<u>13</u>
<u>14</u>	<u>15</u>	16	17	18	19	<u>20</u>
21	<u>22</u>	23	24	25	26	27
28	29*	30*				

Predicting Ovulation in a 32-Day Cycle

NOVEMBER

	1*	2*	3*	4*	5*	6
7	8	9	10	11	12	13
14	15	16	<u>17</u>	<u>18</u>	<u>19</u>	20
21	22	23	24	25	26	27
28	29	30				

DECEMBER

			1	2	3*	4*
5*	6*	7*	8	9	10	11
12	13	14	15	16	17	18
<u>19</u>	<u>20</u>	<u>21</u>	22	23	24	25
26	27	28	29	30	31	

* Menstrual flow.
__ Possible days of ovulation.

ses," which falls in the middle of a twenty-eight-day cycle only. Again I emphasize that the more regular portion of the cycle is the postovulatory portion, that is, between the time of ovulation and the onset of menstruation. There is considerable variation in when ovulation occurs. In many perfectly normal women, it is—regularly or even irregularly—delayed by a week or two, sometimes even more. And, at least in some rare cases, an egg can even be released in the days just after the end of the menstrual flow. But once ovulation does occur, it triggers the series of events that *almost* always culminates in the beginning of menstruation after fourteen or fifteen days—unless, of course, impregnation has occurred.

The examples shown demonstrate how to go about detecting the fertile period in twenty-eight-day and thirty-two-day cycles. But prediction of ovulation on the basis of the calendar method alone is not precise enough. It is useful in getting a general idea of the days of maximal fertility—those in which conception is most likely to occur—but it is a very crude method for pinpointing ovulation with the accuracy necessary to influence sex outcome.

WITH A THERMOMETER

With the third method, you can also take advantage of the fact that, before and after the release of the ovum, the female body undergoes some biological changes which you can learn to detect.

Because of the fluctuation in hormone levels, there are alterations in body temperature. If a woman plots out her temperature throughout her whole cycle, she will find it is relatively low during the first two phases (menstruation and prior to ovulation), dips slightly in some instances, then suddenly goes up a few tenths of a degree or more. This rise in body temperature is due to the presence of progesterone in the blood. Remember, since progesterone appears in significant quantities only *after* ovulation, a relatively high temperature is very good evidence that ovulation has already occurred. (Progesterone injections in males will also produce a temperature rise.)

Because body temperature normally fluctuates during waking hours, sometimes as much as two degrees or more, the only accurate technique for comparing daily changes is by recording what is known as the *basal body temperature,* or BBT. Body temperature normally falls during sleep, and the BBT is the temperature reading *immediately upon waking,* just before it begins to rise after a night of normal restful sleep. This means you must take it *before* you get out of bed, read the paper, have a cup of coffee, or even before you decide to stay put for a while and catch an extra forty winks. (This is why, if you've ever been hospitalized, a nurse interrupts your dreams at some preposterous hour by ramming a thermometer into your mouth.)

Using a form like the one on page 146, the temperature is recorded as a dot for each day, with Day One as the first day of menstruation. The dots are then connected into a simple line graph. Most drugstores carry the charts and special basal thermometers for added ease in detecting small shifts. But regular thermometers are fine for this purpose. If you have difficulty reading a standard type, you might try one of the new digital thermometers.

Either an oral or a rectal thermometer may be used. The rectal is reputed to be slightly more accurate, but the oral is infinitely more convenient and is sufficiently accurate for the purpose. Do keep at least one extra on hand; they are prone to fly across the room at inopportune moments. And in case you must switch thermometers in mid-cycle, be sure the new one has been "standardized" with the previous one, that is, check ahead of time to see that the replacement thermometer gives *exactly* the same reading as the one you've been using so that it will conform to the previous figures. If it does not, you will have to "correct" the readings for the remainder of the current cycle. To clarify, if the new thermometer reads a tenth of a degree higher compared to the old, you should record the readings a tenth of a degree lower. Once you begin a new cycle, no changes are necessary since the readings will all be from the same thermometer.

Set your alarm five minutes early, if necessary, so that you have time to keep the thermometer inserted under your tongue (assuming it is an oral type) for a full three minutes before you do anything else.

You can purchase the chart forms separately or, if you prefer, it shouldn't take more than sixty seconds to copy the sample onto half a sheet of plain graph paper. It is *not* recommended that you simply record the numbers on a sheet of paper because it is difficult to visualize the actual curve that results from comparatively small changes. If you miss a day for whatever reason—becuse you overslept, or were wakened early with an extended pre-dawn phone call, or simply because you forgot—just leave that day blank. A "late" reading is useless for these purposes.

Sources vary somewhat, but the usual "low" readings during the first part of the cycle generally range between 97.2 and 97.8. The temperature *usually* dips slightly on the day of ovulation but this may happen between BBT readings so that you may never be aware of it. The *day after* ovulation the temperature rises by between 0.4 and 1.0 to a "high" in the usual range of about 98.4 to 98.6. While this is considered by some professionals as a dramatic shift, the term is relative. Sometimes the temperature will rise slowly, in "staircase" fashion, causing the fertile days to be less obvious (unfortunately).

The high level is sustained until the beginning of the next menstrual period, at which time the temperature again drops and the cycle starts over. If the period doesn't begin at its usual time and the BBT remains high after two and a half weeks, it's a sure sign of pregnancy.

BBT graphs are particularly useful in natural family planning efforts because a continued temperature rise means that the risk of pregnancy is practically zero (assuming, of course, that you're not pregnant already). The trick for couples seeking pregnancy, when they are following a specific coital timing pattern with respect to ovulation, is *predicting* the egg's release. Women often ask me, "How do you know the temperature has dipped until it has already dipped?" The answer is that you can't be absolutely sure, but with records from a few months you generally do see a pattern emerge.

Although there is not full consensus, the experts for the most part agree that ovulation takes place the day before the sustained rise in temperature. (A few professionals have placed it at two days prior to the rise, but one day is more commonly accepted.) Since nature tends to be regular, *most* women will ovulate around the same day of each menstrual cycle. If you happen to be one of the few whose cycles are regularly irregular, you may wish to consult your gynecologist about regulating it temporarily with the use of hormones, but I recommend it only on a "last resort" basis. Aside from the fact that the medication is very expensive, most physicians today are extremely conservative in the use

Examples of Changes in Basal Body Temperature When Ovulation Has Occurred

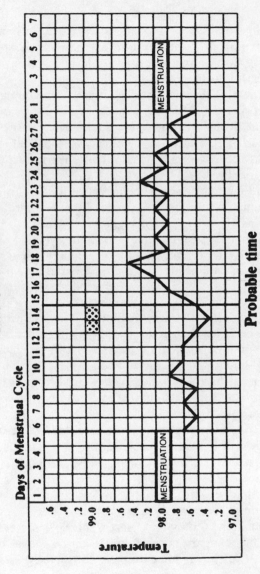

Days of Menstrual Cycle

Temperature

Probable time of ovulation

Examples of Changes in Basal Body Temperature When Ovulation Has Not Occurred

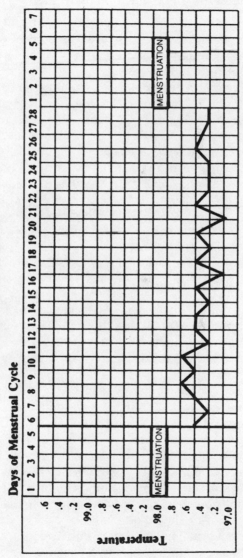

of hormone therapy for any reason. While it is unlikely
to be harmful in any way over a period of only two or
three months, you should discuss the relevant factors
with your doctor.

Even for regular cycles, temperature charts are often
criticized as too erratic for practical use. But more
often it is the lifestyle rather than the temperature
curve that is erratic. The BBT is intended to be the
reading after *a full night of normal restful sleep,* since
the temperature reaches its lowest level only after all
muscular and mental activity has ceased for several
hours. If you frequently keep late hours, suffer from
insomnia, or have your sleep periodically interrupted
for any reason, you decrease your chances for consistent readings in either the low or high phases. Other
interfering factors include such "unavoidables" as
colds, gastrointestinal distress, and emotional upsets;
and at least one avoidable one; alcoholic beverages.
This doesn't mean you can't enjoy a cocktail or two
before dinner or during the evening; it's immoderate
indulgence that plays havoc, usually in more ways than
simple body temperature. (When you're trying to become pregnant, as well as throughout pregnancy, two
should be your limit anyway.)

It's wise to make a note on your chart of any circumstance which might cause deviation from that night of
"restful normal sleep" or which might possibly influence body temperature in some other way, such as any
medication that you do not normally take. After three
or four months this added information will help determine more accurately what your usual temperature
cycle is—or should be.

Above all, be patient. Don't become discouraged
after the first month or two because the charts don't

seem to be telling you anything. In all likelihood they probably will, *if* you are following directions carefully.

BY OBSERVING CHANGES IN MUCUS

Finally, you can get some clues aboout ovulation timing by observing changes in the cervical mucus that is released through the vagina.

This mucus responds to hormones. During most of the cycle, the cervix, or opening to the uterus, is blocked with a plug of cells. Sperm, or potentially infectious agents, cannot enter the uterus. Just before ovulation, when the level of the hormone estrogen is increasing, this mucus plug begins to disintegrate, creating a gradual whitish discharge into the vagina. This outpouring is called *mucorrhea,* and it usually begins about five or six days before ovulation. By the day of ovulation, the mucus produced by the cervical glands is particularly clear and profuse and has a unique characteristic termed *Spinnbarkeit,* a German word meaning "threadability." At or just before ovulation this discharge can be stretched, much like a piece of highly elastic dough.

Just as an aside here, it was increased understanding of the changes in the cervical mucus that led to one of our new forms of birth control, the "mini-pill." These tablets contain an artificial form of progesterone that seems to act directly on the mucus, causing it to retain its pluglike characteristic, thus blocking sperm from entering the uterus. One problem, though, is that the mucus is so sensitive to hormones that forgetting even one or two pills can weaken the plug enough for sperm to get in.

By keeping aware of the cervical discharge, a woman can extract considerable information about the timing of ovulation. The usual pattern goes like this: The days of menstrual bleeding will be followed by a number of "dry days." Then there will be a few "wet days," when a cloudy, sticky secretion can be noted. Finally, about two to three days before ovulation, the mucus will become thin (by this time it is 98 percent water), clear, slippery, and "stretchable," and will look much like raw egg white. There may also be a less marked increase in mucorrhea two to three days before the menstrual period, because of a minor rise in estrogen at that point in the cycle.

The succession of changes may not be so noticeably clear-cut in all women, but the discharge will always be watery, clear and profuse at ovulation. The thicker and more sparse it is, the farther you are from its occurrence.

Once ovulation takes place and progesterone is in command, the cervical mucus presents an almost impenetrable barrier of thick material. Very few, if any, spermatozoa can get into the tubes at this time. Indeed, a method of family planning based exclusively on detection of the wet (fertile) and dry (sterile) days has been proposed by Drs. John and Evelyn Billings, Australian authorities on the rhythm method and authors of such natural family planning guides as *The Ovulation Method*. Field tests of this method are being carried out in several parts of the world. Its value in pinpointing the most fertile days in a given cycle is undisputed; for purposes of sex selection, the "mucus method" is even more useful. In addition to indicating the ovulation day itself, it also "announces" the *pre*-ovulatory period. As we shall see in a moment, this advance notice can be of crucial importance in scheduling intercourse that will favor conception of a specific sex.

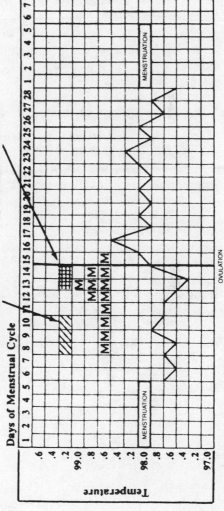

"Boy" and "Girl" Days for Conceptions Occurring as a Result of Sexual Intercourse
(Twenty-eight-day cycle used as example)

Increased probability of a male birth

Increased probability of a female birth

Days of Menstrual Cycle

MENSTRUATION

MENSTRUATION

OVULATION

Temperature

M = mucus discharge

The chart on the previous page gives you an idea of what the mucus discharge pattern in relation to the temperature graph might look like. Remember that the preovulatory portion of this chart will be longer or shorter if the cycle is longer or shorter than twenty-eight days.

It's Not as Difficult as It May Seem

If you've skimmed through this chapter too quickly, you're probably sitting there right now wondering if there isn't an easier way to determine ovulation time. Landrum Shettles thinks there is. He claims that Tes-Tape—chemically treated paper strips used by diabetics to test for urine sugar—will turn its darkest color just before ovulation. But Shettles seems to be the only person who thinks so. I have been unable to find any other informed professional who supports his contention.

If the methods I have outlined seem complicated, it's only because they are new to you. After you've taken a little time to become more familiar with them, you'll realize they're far simpler than they appear to most people at first encounter.

In the next chapter we'll take a look at how these techniques can be used to your advantage.

5

Beating Those 50-50 Odds: How to Increase Your Chances in Sex Selection Roulette

Now it's time to put your new-found knowledge to work. By now you undoubtedly realize that the essential step toward swaying those 50-50 odds is determining your probable day of ovulation. Since, as we have seen, that can sometimes be a bit tricky, I recommend that you utilize all of the established techniques. Even if your menstrual cycles are extremely regular, the procedures act to cross-check each other.

Identifying the Boy and Girl Days

There are three methods of identifying boy and girl days.

THE BASAL BODY TEMPERATURE CURVE

A woman using this method must take her temperature every day upon awakening, starting at the end of the menstrual flow (but counting the first day of the flow as Day One), as described in the last chapter. Remember that if you're in the middle of breakfast when you realize the thermometer is still on the night table, it's too late to use it that day.

After a few months, unless you have a very irregular cycle, you'll have a good idea of how many days elapse between the beginning of a cycle and the rise in temperature which indicates that ovulation has occurred. (Again I admonish you to be patient. Some things just can't be hurried.)

If you want a boy, have sexual relations on the sixth, fifth, and fourth days before the expected day of the temperature rise, and avoid sex, or if you prefer use a mechanical form of contraception, until three days after the temperature rise. If you do not conceive in the first three cycles of trying, you might move the schedule to the "right" one day—have coitus on the fifth, fourth, and third days before the expected rise in temperature. But keep in mind that by the time you reach the third day, you're closely approaching the "girl days." There are also indications that abstention from all intercourse for several days before these "boy days" will help increase your chances of conceiving sooner because the total sperm count is likely to be higher.

If you want a girl, eliminate sex until two or three days before the expected rise in temperature. To avoid the problems that may accompany the fertilization of an "old" egg, *do not* have sexual intercourse without contraception on the day or two immediately following ovulation. Once the temperature has been level for one day, there is no need for further precautions. Ovulation has already taken place and there is almost no risk of pregnancy.

"WET DAYS" AND "DRY DAYS"

Over the course of a few months, take note of the changes in vaginal secretions. These will give you a clue to the onset of ovulation. As I mentioned, the observation of mucus as a means of predicting ovulation is now widely used by couples practicing natural methods of birth control, and because this method may have some practical application to your sex predetermination efforts, I'll present some of the details on its use.

In the days following the end of the menstrual flow (possibly some six or more days before ovulation), the *infertile* mucus appears. It is sticky, cloudy and glue-like. Some two or three days before ovulation, you will notice the *fertile* mucus, the clear, slippery, wet discharge that stretches without breaking. Record these changes on your temperature chart (see illustration on the next page).

There is significant variation from woman to woman in the timing and quantity of mucorrhea, so take the time to learn for yourself how many days elapse between the first vaginal secretions and the rise in body temperature. Generally speaking, sexual intercourse during the so-called infertile mucus days (if that is the same as six, five or four days before the shift in body temperature) will increase the chances of conceiving a male child. Intercourse during the fertile mucus days (one or two days before the shift) will increase the chances of conceiving a female child.

Mucorrhea (Cervical Secretions) During the Menstrual Cycle

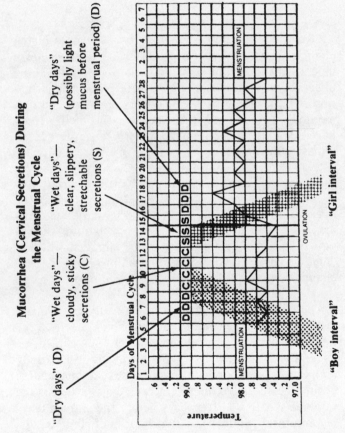

"Dry days" (D)

"Wet days"— cloudy, sticky secretions (C)

"Wet days"— clear, slippery, stretchable secretions (S)

"Dry days" (possibly light mucus before menstrual period) (D)

156

CALENDAR PREDICTIONS

If the temperature and secretion-analysis methods sound too complicated to you, a calendar may be of some help in predicting boy and girl days, particularly if you have a regular menstrual cycle. But keep in mind that calendar methods are only a crude means of predicting ovulation. They generally give just a rough idea of when the most "pregnancy prone" days will occur. Remembering that ovulation takes place approximately fourteen days before the menstrual flow begins, you might make the following calculations on a twenty-eight-day cycle:

			DECEMBER		probable time of ovulation	
(boy days)					(girl days)	
1*	2*	3*	4*	5*	6	7
8	9	10	11	12	13	14
15	16	17	18	19	20	21
22	23	24	25	26	27	28
29*	30*	31*				

* Menstrual flow.

All the scientific evidence gathered up to now points to the conclusion that you will significantly raise your odds on having a child of the sex of your choice by following one of these insemination timing patterns. Again, we are talking of an increase from the normal 50 percent odds on a boy birth to up to 68 percent with early-cycle insemination, and for a girl to about 56 or 57 percent when insemination takes place near ovulation.

If you describe this method to parents who claim to be familiar with the exact timing of their children's conception, a good proportion of them undoubtedly will contradict you and the method. They and we could both be right. Remember, if in early-cycle inseminations 68 percent of the babies are male, that means that 32 percent are female. This method sways the odds in your favor. It does not rule out the possibility of the other sex.

Does This Timing Procedure Really Work?

The coital timing procedures presented in this chapter are based on international studies of both artificially and naturally inseminated women. The "68 percent male" figure is derived from analyses of 1,318 pregnancies (875 couples following the rhythm method and conceiving naturally, some as a result of planning a pregnancy, some as a result of accidental pregnancies; and 443 artificial insemination cases). Initially the largest study ever carried out in this area, the findings have since found support in other research. (For those who would like to read more technical accounts of the research, citations of recent medical journal articles on sex ratio and timing of intercourse are included in the Selected References at the back of this book.) Most studies in the area of sex selection are considerably smaller because of the difficulties in obtaining such data. Couples do not routinely record either when they have sexual intercourse or the woman's temperature upon awaking. Nor is it easy to persuade a couple to dispense this type of information for "the sake of science." Natural family planners—who *are* motivated— are an ideal group to study because they do routinely have this information, but they are not available in unlimited numbers.

I emphasize that the Guerrero observations are the first to be based on statistics derived from conceptions that result from sexual intercourse. The results have been evaluated by means of standard statistical tests and have been found to be "statistically significant," that is, it is highly unlikely that they occurred by chance.

Is There Any Other Supporting Evidence?

In retrospect, the observation that early-cycle insemination has a higher probability of leading to a male birth is consistent with some other biological and social evidence we have.

First, those early German studies of soldiers and their wives indicating that sex well before ovulation led to a greater than expected ratio of boy babies were probably correct. But so were the statistics on artificial insemination which revealed just the opposite results (see the table on pages 164–66.) It appears that the type of insemination as well as the timing is important here. All but one study of human sex ratios by time of natural insemination show that early-cycle inseminations favor male births. The percentage of male births early in the cycle ranged from 60 to 84 percent. In the one deviant study (by Dr. Benendo) ovulation was not determined in a precise manner. All human studies of artificial insemination have indicated that there is a surplus of male births at the time of ovulation as measured by the thermal shift. Again, the one initially discrepant study was by Dr. Cohen, and when it was reanalyzed by a standard methodology that difference disappeared.

All animal studies that we know of show a higher

proportion of males conceived at the beginning of the reproductive cycle (far from ovulation) when animals mate normally, but when they are artificially inseminated it is the inseminations at ovulation that yield more males (see the table on page 167).

Why should there be such a drastic difference depending on the circumstances under which conception takes place? Certainly research would be much less complicated if both types of insemination, artificial and natural, followed the same pattern. Right now we do not know the answer for certain, but there is good reason to suspect that various biochemical changes which occur in the female body during intercourse, but not during artificial insemination, may be responsible. For instance, the secretions in the vagina and the cervix may change during coitus in a way that may influence either the boy- or girl-producing sperm (we'll look at this in detail later in the chapter). Moreover, it is obvious that sperm have a different "starting point." In artificial insemination semen is placed close to the cervix; when they enter the body in sexual intercourse they have to work their own way up the vagina.

The fact that we cannot yet explain exactly why sex outcomes are exactly the opposite for the two kinds of insemination should not lead us to deny that there is an important association here. To do so would be like denying that a woman is pregnant just because the father isn't known. The observation is clear. The explanation for it may come much later.

Second, as Dr. William H. James, of the Department of Biometry, University College, London, has noted, if the timing of insemination does have an impact on the sex outcome of the baby, then fraternal twins—that is, those children who develop from two different eggs—

should be more likely to be of the same sex than of opposite sexes. This assumes that both eggs are released from the ovary and fertilized at about the same time, a generally accepted assumption.

And indeed this is true. Fraternal twins *are* more likely to be of the same sex, very possibly because vaginal conditions at the time when insemination occurs are the same for both sperm. If the timing of insemination did not make any difference, you would expect to see half the pairs of fraternal twins the same sex, half of different sexes. (The reason, of course, is that the same 50-50 ratio would hold true just as if the two fertilized eggs were in two different women, or in the same woman at two different times.)

Third, we can explain many of the "social" differences in sex ratio by examining variations in the timing of insemination. For instance, we know that the proportion of male births rises during and just after wars. (Some have said that this is God's way of replacing men lost in battle.) Very possibly this is due to the fact that soldiers home on leave or just reentering civilian life have sexual intercourse *more frequently* than they would under other circumstances. And logically, frequency would be a factor, given our observation that the boy days come earlier in the cycle than the girl days.

Frequent intercourse increases the possibility of having a male child simply because one hits the boy days first. For example, if a couple has intercourse five times a month, it might be on days 6, 13, 18, 25, and 27. The probability of having coitus on the male-oriented early-cycle days is considerably less for this couple than for a couple having sexual relations every other day— perhaps days 5, 7, 9, 11, 13, and so on. The mere fact that the "boy interval" comes first means that frequent intercourse favors a male child.

Similarly, this explanation can be applied to the observation that young couples—those conceiving their first child, those recently married—have more boys. Here too frequency may be the critical factor. Perhaps the fact that more male births are recorded in the month of June than in any other month can be explained by the fact that as the temperature goes down (nine months earlier, in September) the coital frequency may go up.

Orthodox Jews offer interesting case material in evaluating the effect of insemination timing on the sex outcome of the child, because religious law governs their sexual intercourse pattern. Specifically, the *niddah* (separation) regulations forbid coitus (or any other male-female contact) for seven full days after the termination of the menstrual flow. That would place the first allowable coitus around day 12 or 13, which, according the Guerrero theory, would mean that Orthodox Jews would have more than the average percentage of girls. Dr. James recently tested that hypothesis by analyzing official birth statistics in Israel (a country that distinguishes between Jewish and non-Jewish births) and found that the Jewish couples *do* have slightly fewer male children. What proportion of Israel's Jewish population practices *niddah* is not known. I suspect that if those who strictly follow this aspect of the religious code were analyzed separately, an even higher preponderance of daughters would be found.

Reports in the press, as well as in earlier sex selection books and at least one current study, to the effect that Orthodox Jews have fewer female children is very possibly the result of incomplete reporting. Since many

Orthodox Jewish families have a very strong preference for males, and the birth registration system in small religious sects is not always precise, many female births may simply go unreported.

There is another explanation for this apparent contradiction, however. In 1979, Susan Harlap of the Hebrew University of Jerusalem (supported by a contract from the Center for Population Research of the National Institute of Child Health and Human Development in Bethesda) conducted a study of 3,658 births among Jewish women practicing *niddah*. She noted that resumption of intercourse is frequently delayed a few days for various reasons and thus may not take place at all until after ovulation. While the study revealed a higher proportion of male births, Harlap notes that the highest proportion occurred as a result of conceptions *two days after ovulation*. Further, the lowest proportion were from conceptions on or near the day of ovulation—in accordance with Guerrero's "girl days." This observation also supports other research that male births tend to predominate in postovulatory conceptions.

However, as I have noted elsewhere, there is also a great deal of evidence that this is the worst possible time to begin a pregnancy; in fact, I am unaware of any scientist or other professional who advocates such timing, in a deliberate sense, for any reason. Most distinctly advise against it.

Sex Selection Theories in Conflict?

I have emphasized in this section and elsewhere that the latest timing advice for sex selection is the opposite

Summary of the Published Accounts of the Influence of Time of Insemination on the Human Sex Ratio

Type	Time of Insemination	Sex Ratio	Comments	Author, Year Published
Natural	Days of menstrual cycle	More males the first ten days	Very few cases	Swift, 1878
Natural	Days of menstrual cycle	More males the first ten days	Time of insemination from records of military leave	Pryll, 1916
Natural	Days of menstrual cycle	More males the first ten days		Bolaffio, 1922
Natural	Days of menstrual cycle	More males the first ten days	Time of insemination from records of military leave	Asdell, 1927
Natural	Days of menstrual cycle	More males early in cycle, specifically, five or more days before ovulation		Guerrero, 1968, 1970, 1974

164

Natural	Days of menstrual cycle	More males early in the cycle	Inference from sex distribution of fraternal twins	James, 1971
Natural	Time around ovulation	More males the day before ovulation	Ovulation not determined in precise manner	Benendo, 1970
Natural	Expected onset of menstruation minus 14 days	Fewer males near day of ovulation; more males in previous one or two days; high percentage of males two days after ovulation	Study of 3658 infants of Jewish women practicing *niddah*	Harlap, 1979
Artificial	Related to B.B.T.	More males around thermal shift	These are observations on which Shettles method is based	Kleegman, 1954
Artificial	Related to B.B.T.	More males around thermal shift		Yoshida, 1960

Summary of the Published Accounts of the Influence of Time of Insemination on the Human Sex Ratio (continued)

Type	Time of Insemination	Sex Ratio	Comments	Author, Year Published
Artificial	Related to mucorrhea	No significant difference noted around ovulation, but when date reanalyzed by RG using standard methodology, more males around the shift		Cohen, 1967
Artificial	Time around ovulation	More males with fresh semen "in agreement with the reports of Guerrero"; fewer males cryostored (frozen) sperm	Very large, retrospective study; time of insemination not precise	Martinez & Richardson, 1982

Summary of the Published Accounts of the Influence of Time of Mating on the Sex Ratio of Different Animals

Animal	Time of Insemination	Sex Ratio	Type of Insemination	Year Published
Cow	Early vs. late estrus	Early: more males Late: more females	Natural	1917
Rat	Early vs. late estrus	Early: more males Late: more females	Natural	1925
Rat	Early vs. late estrus	Early: more males Late: more females	Natural	1927
Mouse	Early vs. late estrus	Early: more males Late: more females	Natural	1962
Rat	Early vs. late estrus	Early: more females Late: more males	Artificial	1941
Cow	Early vs. late estrus	Early: more females	Artificial	1970
Rabbit	Before and after ovulation	More males until ovulation, sudden decrease after	Unclear, possibly artificial	1934

from that of earlier books on the subject. But it is worthwhile noting here *that there is no conflict whatever between this new scientific knowledge about the timing of intercourse and the offspring's sex* and the information gathered during the 1960s. That early theory was based on artificial insemination. The new data fully support those observations: more males *are* born when artificial insemination takes place very close to ovulation. The only thing Dr. Guerrero and others now object to (and it's an important objection) is that the artificial insemination data were assumed to be applicable to couples conceiving in sexual intercourse. We have evidence now that this is not true. New investigations have served to confirm earlier observations—and expand knowledge—by offering the first evidence on natural insemination.

Dr. Shettles and David Rorvik in their book, *Choose Your Baby's Sex,* attempt to make Guerrero's observations about artificial insemination compatible with their timing advice by explaining that their techniques, based on coital positions and precoital douching, *simulate* the conditions of artificial insemination and thus yield the same results as that type of insemination. But there is no reason to believe this is true. The biological changes that occur (or, more likely, don't occur) in a woman's body during the artificial insemination process in a physician's office cannot be "simulated" in the bedroom.

Public interest in sex selection has evoked a great many articles on the subject in both the popular media and professional journals. Unfortunately, their authors often fail to emphasize—or sometimes even to mention—the profound difference between the results of natural and artificial insemination. This has unavoid-

ably created a great many confused readers and prospective parents who feel they are caught in the middle
of an "us vs. them" battlefield, when in fact this is not
the case.

In comparing earlier views on sex selection and the
timing of intercourse with that presented here, you
might consider that by following the Shettle-Rorvik
advice in the hopes of having a girl baby you would
drastically reduce your chances, because you'd be concentrating coitus three or more days before ovulation,
on what we have found are the "boy days." You might
thus be reducing your naturally given fifty-fifty odds of
having a girl to 32 percent, because early-cycle insemination yields up to 68 percent male births. New research shows that at the time of ovulation the odds on
having a female are about 57 percent, which obviously
means that the odds on a male birth would be 43
percent. Thus, by following the Shettles method for a
boy, you would reduce your odds from the natural fifty-
fifty to 43 percent. In either case, by following a methodology based on the results of artificial insemination
you are reducing your odds on having a child of the sex
of your choice.

In all fairness, I should mention that Guerrero's data
have occasionally been criticized because temperature
charts are not always a reliable indicator of ovulation.
The point would be valid were it not for the considerable size of the study. In a sampling of that many
subjects, it can be assumed that "errors" of that nature
would cancel themselves out. In other words, there's
no reason to believe that possible miscalculations on a
temperature chart would consistently favor one sex
over the other.

A Caveat

Sex selection using coital timing techniques would be a relatively easy method if there were an equal probability of conceiving on the days before ovulation. But there is not.

What comes as a surprise to many couples who have been practicing birth control for many years is that planned conceptions do not always occur "on schedule" immediately after stopping contraception. This is especially true after oral contraception is discontinued, when at least the first two cycles are likely to be highly irregular and ovulation may not occur at all. This is not surprising when you know that "the Pill" functions by interfering with normal hormone production, which may take a little time to re-establish itself. Occasionally, gynecologists will prescribe synthetic hormones in order to jolt the reproductive system back into its usual routine.

Statistical studies have shown that the probability of conception rises with the frequency of sexual intercourse (not a remarkable observation!). If you have random sexual relations five times during the month—that is, you do not try to either avoid or "hit" ovulation—you will have a 16 percent chance of conceiving in the first month. This percentage "success" rate for the first month will rise to about 32 percent if you have intercourse twelve times a month. All of this, of course, assumes that both partners are fully fertile.

If, on the other hand, you are trying to conceive, but without using any sex selection techniques, and you make an effort to schedule sexual relations around the time of ovulation, you increase your odds on a pregnancy in the first month to between 26 percent (with intercourse five times) and 45 percent (twelve times).

Although you will raise your odds on a male birth by having sexual intercourse well before ovulation, you should realize that this is *not* the most "fertile" portion of the cycle, and as a result it could take a number of months—possibly five to eight—to conceive, even if you have frequent intercourse on the "boy days" and you are both fertile. It is markedly simpler to plan a girl birth, since the "girl days" coincide with the period of maximum fertility.

The fact that the boy days fall in the less fertile portion of the menstrual cycle should be taken into account by couples who are eager to have a child quickly and/or have experienced infertility problems in the past. For instance, one couple I counseled (the husband was thirty-eight, the wife thirty-four) had been trying to conceive for two years. Both had undergone infertility examinations, but no specific problem could be identified. The infertility specialist had told them to "keep trying." They had their hearts set on having one child, a son. But I had to advise them against following this regimen for a male child, because it would only increase their odds of never having children. A couple with a nonspecific fertility problem should have sexual intercourse frequently in the days just before ovulation. (There is a possible alternative: A man and woman who strongly desire a son may wish to consider artificial insemination with the new sperm separation techniques. This will be covered in more detail in the next chapter.)

Coital Timing and Offspring's Sex: What Do These Discoveries Mean?

Obviously there must be some underlying biological reasons why timing of insemination within the menstrual cycle is an important variable in human sex determination, and why women who are artificially inseminated have more sons than those who have intercourse right at the time of ovulation. As I suggested earlier, one possible explanation is biochemical in nature—that is, maybe there is something unique about the female reproductive tract early in the cycle that is favorable to male-producing sperm. If this is so, perhaps in addition to following the timing pattern, you can take steps to make the vaginal and cervical areas more receptive to one or the other type of sperm.

Sex Outcome and Chemistry

As I've discussed, the theory that alkalinity—whether from douching with an alkaline preparation, like baking soda and water, or from female orgasm preceding male ejaculation—favors male births has been around for decades, and, in the case of the orgasm theory, for centuries. But there simply is no proof that this theory is valid. On the contrary, as I mentioned earlier, the latest evidence points to the fact that it is *invalid*.

We know that semen itself dramatically neutralizes the pH of the vagina. Most specialists consider it unlikely that douching beforehand could either enhance or overpower the semen's effect. A research team at Yale School of Medicine, using laboratory procedures to "race" male- and female-producing sperm in various chemical solutions, concluded: "It appears unlikely that X and Y sperm can be differentiated on the basis of migration through fluids of varying pH's." Instead they found that both boy- and girl-producing sperm moved most freely in alkaline environments that were approximately the same as that of the cervical mucus at the time of ovulation. These same results have been duplicated by other investigators during the past few years.

But in spite of all the evidence, or rather the lack of it, the acid-alkaline theory makes sense in terms of what we know about the timing of intercourse and the sex of the baby. We know that the vagina and the cervix undergo chemical changes in response to female hormones. Early in the cycle the vagina is relatively alkaline; as ovulation approaches, it become more acid, relatively less alkaline. The cervical secretions show just the opposite pattern: they become more alkaline— that is, less hostile to sperm—as ovulation approaches. If it is true that male-producing sperm survive better in alkaline environments, this would explain why they have a better chance both in the less alkaline vagina early in the cycle in the natural insemination, and right at ovulation when they are placed at the alkaline cervical opening during artificial insemination.

A number of scientists now feel that the original theory proposed by Dr. Unterberger back in the 1930s should be reevaluated. The flurry of experiments that followed (under the auspices of the *Daily News* and others) generally dealt with animals and often used artificial insemination techniques. No one (as far as I am aware) has ever studied a large group of women who tried precoital douching with alkaline solutions. And it seems that no one has ever studied the effects of the acid douching on probabilities of having a girl baby. Unterberger and others explained (although it is difficult to believe) that they never had a patient who felt strongly enough about having a daughter to try their method.

Similarly, and perhaps more importantly, we should look more closely at the chemical changes of female orgasm to see if orgasm-induced alterations in vaginal and cervical secretions have any effect on sperm.

IN THE MEANTIME . . .

It is difficult for me to endorse a technique that has been hammered down by legitimate scientific research. Nevertheless, I continue to feel there is still much to be learned about the biochemistry of the reproductive system. While *laboratory* study may rule out pH as a factor influencing sexual outcome, we do not really know that this absolutely rules out any effect it might have in a *human* environment. Perhaps pH acts in conjunction with some other, still unknown, factor that tends to favor either the X's or the Y's according to fluctuating conditions.

Mild douches of both baking soda and vinegar are harmless and, as I have already explained, the "recipes" do coincide with the changing environment of the vagina as the cycle shifts from boy days to girl days. In view of this "presumptive" evidence, it certainly isn't going to hurt anything to enhance the conditions by douching, if you wish to do so. Although we don't yet understand why, the possibility remains that douching before sexual intercourse and planning (or avoiding) female orgasm during the appropriate baby days *may* boost your chances for the preferred sex above the 68 or 56–57 percent mark.

If you are hoping for a boy, use a solution of two tablespoons of baking soda to one quart of lukewarm water, within one hour before intercourse. Additionally, attempt to have orgasm well before your husband.

If you are hoping for a girl, prepare a douche with two tablespoons of white vinegar to one quart of lukewarm water and use it within the hour before sexual intercourse. Avoid orgasm on the days in the fertile "girl" period.

There are no standard "prescriptions" for female orgasm; it is a subject very much dominated by personal preference. Presumably *if* (notice the emphasis on *if*) the physiology of female orgasm does in some way favor the migration of Y sperm, managing to have your sexual climax precede your husband's by at least a minute or two *might* give those Y's a head start. If you avoid orgasm, the circumstances *may* favor the X sperm.

The clitoris, the small organ which lies just inside the upper apex of the inner vaginal lips, is probably the female's most erotically responsive area. Usually the clitoral head is about the size of a pea, but during sexual excitement this head as well as the rest of the clitoris becomes somewhat enlarged. Although female orgasm must be preceded by some form of clitoral stimulation, women frequently report that their sex partners often try "too hard." With prolonged direct stimulation, the clitoris becomes extremely sensitive and causes the woman to lose the level of excitement she has attained.

If you have difficulty experiencing orgasm, I suggest you ask a physician to refer you to a sex therapist for the type of instruction that has helped thousands of women with orgasmic problems. (The benefits, of course, reach far beyond the possible influence on your baby's sex.) Additionally, I recommend that you read a book on the psychology and physiology of female sexual climax; a very good one is *Woman's Orgasm* by Georgia Kline-Graber and Benjamin Graber, M.D.

TEMPERATURES, CALENDARS, DOUCHES, MUCORRHEA AND MARRIAGE

In talking about the physiology of sex predetermination, it is easy to forget for a moment that there is more to having a baby—of whatever sex—than Fallopian tubes and temperature readings.

One woman I spoke with who very much wanted a son would work on the forthcoming month's "schedule" the very day her menstrual period began. She would conspicuously circle the boy days and leave a copy of her calendar on her husband's desk, with a carbon on his night table. After about six months they did conceive (and they did have the son they wanted), but the husband confided to me that he had begun to feel like a trained seal.

If you are going to take this timing schedule seriously, be prepared for some rough moments. A husband may be out of town on business on the most important boy day, and it may be impractical to rendezvous at an airport motel in a city midway between for the purpose of insemination. Or a wife may fall asleep early on the night of the long-awaited girl day, and it may not be appropriate to awaken her to perform the rites.

Additionally and understandably, most women are not enthusiastic about interrupting a romantic prelovemaking encounter to grapple with some very unromantic douching equipment. (Most husbands are even less enthusiastic.) And some part of the procedure is quite likely to go wrong. One woman reported that she got the baking soda mixed up with baking powder. When the mixture began to foam like a witch's brew, she got the message. Another told me with frustration about the evening the girl day arrived. She had carefully prepared her vinegar and water solution, slipped into a sexy negligee and then into the bathroom—only to have her douching equipment explode all over her and the sexy negligee.

Another couple confided to me that it was more than a little embarrassing for them when *the* day arrived while they were staying with friends out of town and they had to ask the hostess for a cup of vinegar before they retired.

Sex determination efforts, like infertility regimens that try to pinpoint ovulation, can prove tedious. Be prepared to break at least two or three thermometers before you succeed. Certainly the motivation must be there if your attempts are going to work, and it's best to keep good-humored about all your efforts.

But there are some rewards that go with the rigors of keeping track of temperature, watching for cervical mucus changes, and being alert to other signs in the menstrual system. One is the benefit of increased self-knowledge. Some couples I've talked to seem afraid of their bodies; they don't understand how reproduction works and they are embarrassed about the specifics. By developing a sophistication about the intricacies of the menstrual cycle and accepting them as normal, natural, and in a sense miraculous in their regularity and precision, you may find that many previous anxieties are alleviated. You will inevitably become self-conscious—in a positive sense—of the delicate biological clockwork which leads to the conception of a child, and may well acquire a fuller sense of respect for yourself, your body and its potential.

There is at least one additional advantage in recording morning temperatures. If the basal body temperature remains elevated for sixteen or more days after ovulation, it is one of the earliest, simplest, and most reliable of "natural" pregnancy tests. As a graph in the next section shows, a missed period with elevated temperature indicates pregnancy.

Although the "how to" of sex selection is our topic here, I think it is worthwhile to cover two subjects which may be of interest if you do become pregnant (pregnancy testing) and if you don't (infertility). "Family planning" is a broad term. Attempts to achieve pregnancy and to choose the sex of your child should be put into a broader context.

Pregnancy Tests

If you were practicing birth control for some time before you made the decision to have a child, you will probably frequently think about the fact that you *could* become pregnant during the very first month. But beware. You may be also too self-aware, and may begin to find "pregnancy symptoms" that aren't there.

It is theoretically possible, of course, that you could "just know" you're pregnant the very night it happens—or within a few days after you've missed your period. Some women get early clues that they are pregnant; not only is their menstrual period "late," but their breasts are fuller and more sensitive than they usually are premenstrually, and may even feel vaguely tingling. Morning sickness may occur even within a couple of days after the expected menstrual flow, urination may become more frequent, and the desire to fall asleep even in the middle of the day may be almost overwhelming.

If you become pregnant, you may experience some slight staining for a day or two about the time of the missed period, a form of spotting that results from the new cell's successful attempt to break through the layers of the endometrium.

But the evidence that you are pregnant is not really impressive until your normal menstrual period is ten days to two weeks late. After that point, however, your condition needs some scientific confirmation.

Although it's not a good idea to go running into your physician's office the very moment you even suspect a pregnancy, it is also not wise to wait much more than a couple of weeks after missing a period before having a laboratory assessment.

There are a number of different types of tests, all of which are based on the fact that pregnant women produce the hormone HCG (short for human chorionic gonadotrophin). Up to a few years ago, most such tests were performed by injecting frogs, rabbits, or other animals with specimens of the women's urine. Today's methods are sophisticated enough to bypass the high cost and inconvenience of animal assistance and are instead performed by means of direct chemical analysis of either urine or blood. They also offer the advantage of results within a few hours—remarkable progress in comparison to the original Ascheim-Zondek test (also known as the "A–Z" or "rabbit" test) which required a full forty-eight hours and a slaughtered bunny for diagnosis.

After a shaky beginning, during which all home pregnancy tests were for a time removed from the market, those available in most pharmacies now are fairly reliable. However, there is some tendency toward false negatives (that is the test indicating the patient is not pregnant, when in fact she is), primarily because they utilize the less accurate technique of urine analysis.

For little or no additional cost you can have a more accurate test performed at a private laboratory which will use a sample of blood rather than urine. Of course, you can also have the test performed through your doctor, too, but you should be aware that he/she probably sends out your blood specimen to the same kind of lab you can visit yourself at less expense.

As in any field, some labs are superior to others. You may wish to ask for a recommendation from the Planned Parenthood Federation of America, your local health department, county medical society, or your private physician. But bear in mind that you cannot expect reliable results until *at least* two weeks after your first missed period, and even then there is *no* test that is always 100 percent accurate. In most cases, using direct examination, your gynecologist can detect pregnancy by three weeks after your first missed period. At that very early stage, however, most doctors prefer that a final diagnosis be confirmed by lab examination. (There are numerous cases on record where tumorous growths have mimicked pregnancy in every respect *except* the usual lab test.)

One self-observation technique that indicates pregnancy and should prompt you to see a physician for confirmation simply involves the temperature method. If you are taking your temperature for the purpose of sex selection anyway, just continue the routine in the weeks after ovulation. Again, if your temperature stays up for more than sixteen days after ovulation, the odds are overwhelming that you are pregnant.

The possibility of pregnancy is not the only pressure that should get you to the gynecologist's office after a missed period. On rare occasions, something goes wrong in the days immediately following fertilization.

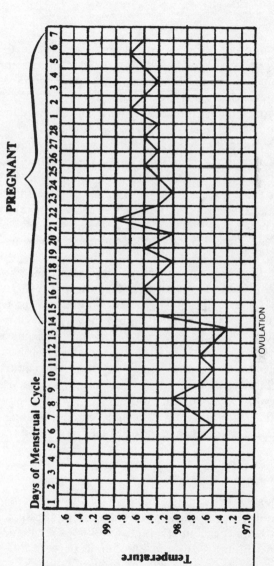

Temperature remaining elevated more than
fourteen days indicates pregnancy.

In about one out of every 300 pregnancies, the fertilized egg implants somewhere other than in the uterus. This "somewhere" could be the ovary, the abdominal cavity or even the cervix, but generally the misplaced zygote settles in the lining of the Fallopian tube and the condition is diagnosed as an *ectopic* (or tubal) *pregnancy*. Perhaps the tube was abnormal in some way and its inner lining didn't do a good enough job in pushing the egg toward its intended destination. But whatever the cause, an ectopic pregnancy poses a serious health risk if it is not detected early. The oviducts just do not have the expansion capability of the uterus—and if the growth is not stopped, the tube will burst.

If you think you may be pregnant, find a gynecologist or family doctor soon, or at least have a test performed. If the test is positive you should set up an immediate appointment with your physician. Don't take unnecessary chances by attempting to diagnose your own condition. Ask some of your friends to recommend a doctor, or if necessary call the local medical society for advice. Your friends can probably give you a more personal evaluation and can clue you in about the physician's orientation, whether he believes in natural childbirth, anesthesia, induced labor, or the stork.

Infertility

For most couples, pregnancy will occur within six to eight months after contraception is omitted. Statistics indicate that 80 percent of couples seeking a pregnancy conceive within a year, and another 10 percent do so within two years. But about 10 percent of couples have problems serious enough to need medical help. In other words, sometimes it just isn't so easy.

In an age when a primary focus is put on technology to prevent births, it comes as a particular shock for a couple to learn that they are physically unable to have children. And usually they can't be really sure that infertility is going to be a problem until they try.

Many things can go wrong between the time sperm are produced and a successfully fertilized ovum implants in the lining of the uterus. Beyond that, there are problems in maintaining a pregnancy once it has occurred.

Before a pregnancy is possible there must be both a healthy egg and a healthy sperm. When a woman seeks help for infertility, her physician will ask her for a few months of basal body temperature graphs. If she has been following this sex selection regimen she will already have those, as well as coital records. It's always a good idea when seeking infertility advice to arrive at the first session with at least three months of basal body temperature records. If you detect a significant inflection in temperature, ovulation may indeed be occurring and the "healthy egg" portion of the formula may be present. Your physician will then probably do a "post-coital" test to learn whether sperm are penetrating the cervical mucus during your fertile period.

A second major portion of an infertility investigation involves checking for healthy (and numerous) sperm. The husband will be asked to submit a semen sample which will be analyzed for sperm count, motility, and the presence of abnormal cells.

If basal body records and/or other procedures indicate that a woman is not ovulating, her physician may recommend hormone treatment to stimulate ovulation. If the husband's sperm count is low he may require hormonal treatment, or possibly a relatively mild form of surgery which leads to improved sperm quality. For instance, if the veins at the side of the testicles become dilated, the production of sperm may be inhibited because of a related rise in temperature. Surgical correction of this condition, known as a varicocle, is reported to improve chances of impregnation. Alternatively, many major cities have "sperm banks" with facilities to freeze a number of semen samples from an infertile man, then concentrate the samples to yield the highest sperm count possible for use in artificially inseminating his wife.

If an egg is released from the ovary, and a sufficient number of sperm are matured in the testes, released into the vagina, and able to make the trip up through the uterus toward the oviducts, fertilization may occur. But then again, maybe it won't. If the tubes are blocked in some way, the egg may not be able to pass through and the sperm may have difficulty getting at the egg; or if the two sex cells do find a way of getting together, the newly formed zygote may not be able to pass through to the uterus. Tubal blockage often results from pelvic inflammation, which may follow, for instance, improperly treated gonorrhea. But it could also be related to another fairly common disease, endometriosis, a condition in which portions of the lining of the uterus travel to and attach to other parts of the pevic region. And often these cells don't just sit there, they grow—possibly on the back of the uterus, around the Fallopian tubes (thus acting as a road block), or around the ovaries.

And if everything goes right up until the time a fertilized ovum enters the uterus, there can still be failure if the endometrium is not adequately prepared. Both estrogen and progesterone should have made the lining of the uterus the ideal place for a fertilized egg to implant and grow. But sometimes that just doesn't happen. A physician may wish to take a small sample of the endometrium for analysis. If he finds that the lining is not so well prepared as it should be at that time of the cycle, he may feel that some form of hormone treatment is in order.

In approximately one-quarter of all normal pregnancies, women experience some type of early bleeding or staining, so this in itself isn't *necessarily* something to worry about. However, another 15 percent of all recognized pregnancies end in miscarriage, or spontaneous abortion, as it is more commonly called during the first three months. (I say "recognized" because doctors know that in addition a great number of spontaneous abortions occur before the women even know they are pregnant, but it is obviously impossible to determine precisely how many.) Abnormality of the fetus accounts for about half of all spontaneous abortions; the other half has so many possible causes that it's difficult, often impossible, to determine the exact reason. A woman who has had more than one miscarriage—certainly if more than two—for no obvious reason should seriously consider consulting an expert in this field.

Returning for a moment to my earlier discussion of overripe eggs, I hope you were aware that I indicated an *increased risk* or problems, which is nowhere near an absolute pronouncement. To begin with, nature doesn't favor fertilization of an old egg. In spite of this, if conception has occurred at this time, there is no need to panic. While there is some chance of trouble ahead, there is a much greater chance there will be none. The recommendation was intended to minimize such risks by cautioning you not to deliberately schedule intercourse within the first couple of days following ovulation, unless you use some type of mechanical contraceptive.

The relatively high incidence of miscarriage is a consideration that should be taken into account in your family planning efforts. On more than one occasion I have had parents come to me in near-hysteria because they had elected to postpone parenthood until the wife was already in her mid-thirites, and then the first pregnancy ended in spontaneous abortion. They feared not only the added delay, but also the possibility that other miscarriages might follow. It really doesn't make much sense to subject yourself to unnecessary stress by waiting too long—especially if your goal is a child of a specific sex—and then expecting events to follow a predetermined timetable. Most of the time, it just doesn't happen that way.

So many things can go wrong that conception and pregnancy may present an unanticipated challenge to some couples. But if you do encounter difficulty, it is likely that, with the help of a competent infertility or gynecology specialist, you'll achieve the pregnancy you're seeking. Keep in mind, however, that a small proportion of couples cannot have children of their own. Some infertile couples turn to artificial insemination, a simple and painless process in which semen is artificially introduced into the vagina shortly before or at the estimated time of ovulation. If the husband is producing some sperm, his semen will be used in artificial insemination. If his sperm count is extremely low, or if no sperm at all can be detected, a donor selected by the physician can contribute a semen sample which may be mixed with the husband's semen. The donor and the receiving woman never learn each other's identity: the whole process is kept as impersonal as a transfusion received from a blood bank. For some couples artificial insemination is the answer to their infertility problems. For others, especially if only donor semen is to be used, there may be significant emotional problems, and adoption may be a more appropriate alternative.

Turning back to our discussion of the "how to" of sex determination, let's now look at the same topic from a different perspective. What if we did have "the" method, one that would offer us a 100 percent effective method of choosing the sex of our children? Would this be a cause for celebration, a major advance in the field of medicine and science, and an unqualified advance in the betterment of mankind—or in this case people-kind? It will be useful to see what the future has in store and to think about the implications of universally available sex determination techniques.

6

Sex Control Methods on the Horizon: Do We Really Want Them?

In January 1922, Julian Huxley told the *New York Herald* that we were rapidly approaching the stage in which it would be possible to control and predict in advance the sex of a child.

As you can see from the description of the current state of knowledge about sex preselection, Huxley was overoptimistic. You *can* now sway the odds in your favor, but you'll still have a wide margin of error.

It is, however, very likely that a nearly 100 percent effective method will be introduced within the next few years. If Huxley were making his prediction today, he would probably be correct. But what he may not have foreseen is that some of the methods carry with them implications that may make many couples think twice about using them.

188

The fact is that there are already methods available professionally that can considerably raise the odds above what I have outlined in this book. But there is a vast difference between what one attempts to achieve within the boundaries of the bedroom and the solicitation of outside assistance. Cost is probably least important in terms of the overall picture. Of far greater significance are the various psychological and ethical implications.

And disappointment is still a risk. After a couple has gone to considerable trouble, expense, and inconvenience in deliberate pursuit of the "right" sex, possible failure might pose serious problems of adjustment.

Perhaps in some future generation, a selective contraceptive—a foam or jelly, a diaphragm with a specially designed filter, or even a pill—will be developed to screen out either the X's or the Y's, but at the moment such notions aren't even close to the drawing board. Theoretically it sounds easy, but when dealing with microscopically small cells, it's a monumental task. The only alternatives now to the do-it-yourself method described in the last chapter are considerably more complicated.

Getting the X (or Y) Out

The most exciting breakthrough in this field is credited to Dr. Ronald J. Ericsson, who has successfully developed a sperm separation technique that is of practical value to men and women desiring a son. Analysis of his corporate records as of September, 1983, reveals a success rate of 77 percent (80 boys out of 104 total pregnancies), a figure that can eventually be expected to climb even higher.

In 1972, Dr. A. M. Roberts of Guy's Hospital Medical School in London, set the wheels in motion when he removed all sperm from a tube of seminal fluid, poured them back in again, and found that Y sperm moved more rapidly through the fluid than did the X sperm. Following up on that discovery, Dr. Ericsson, now president of Gametrics Ltd. in Sausalito, California, and his team began experimenting with various solutions in search of the best one to effectively separate the sperm. The substance had to be thick enough to block the poor swimmers (which include both X's and "substandard" Y's), but not so thick as to hinder good swimmers. After considerable research, serum albumin was found to have the necessary properties.

In the clinical procedure, semen is collected from the male and placed on top of glass columns containing human serum albumin. The sperm then begin swimming toward the bottom of the column "like so many scuba divers." After approximately three hours, the top portion of the column is discarded, and the remainder with its heavy concentration of Y sperm is then injected into the woman by means of artificial insemination.

Using a three-step, three-layer method, the final yield is about 85 to 90 percent Y sperm, representing about 5 percent of the total sperm from the sample. Because the count is so low in the final specimen, more than one attempt may be needed before conception actually occurs. By the same token, the procedure is unlikely to be satisfactory for males who already have a low sperm count.

Unfortunately, as yet there is no comparable method available for producing a girl. The unused portion of the specimen still contains a great many Y's. Even allowing additional time for most of the Y's to swim out, what is left behind contains not only X's, but many deformed and nonmotile Y's, as well as miscellaneous cellular debris—in short, a specimen completely unsuitable for insemination.

Another pioneer in the field, Dr. W. Paul Dmowski, has modified Ericsson's technique at Chicago's Michael Reese Hospital and Medical Center by using only two layers of albumin instead of three. The advantage is greater ease of conception (because fewer sperm are filtered out), but with slightly less complete separation, lowering the odds for a boy to about 70 percent.

Dr. Ericsson's method has been patented and can be used only by doctors who are specially trained and licensed. Gametrics, Ltd., looking toward a bright and busy future, now has branches in ten U.S. cities and four foreign countries, with an additional four foreign branches scheduled to open soon, if they haven't already. (The company also includes an agricultural subsidiary known as The Sperm Firm, designed to improve reproductive efficiency in cattle.)

Concerns have been raised that laboratory "tampering" with sperm could raise the incidence of birth defects. In certain other methods that is a definite risk, but here the very opposite is true simply because the defective sperm tend to be filtered out. Similarly, in a 1979 University of Arkansas study of over 1,000 infants born to mothers who had been artificially inseminated with previously frozen sperm specimens, fewer than one percent suffered from birth defects, compared to 2–6 percent in the general population. (The percentage varies considerably according to which disorders are tabulated as "birth defects.") Additionally, only about half of the usual percentage of miscarriages occurred.

A number of other methods of sperm separation have been under investigation for several years, but with far less success than that of Dr. Ericsson.

One method of separating the two types of cells involves *centrifugation,* literally spinning the semen at high speeds so that the heavier of the two sperm, the X female-producing one, is filtered out. Theoretically, once the X and Y sperm are separated in this fashion the semen fractions can be used in artificial insemination. Some early experiments with animals appear to have been successful in this technique, but very often when semen with predominantly one type of sperm is used, fertility is decreased substantially, and there remains the distinct possibility that the spinning process could damage the sperm, leading to a deformed child or an aborted pregnancy.

Another technique for sperm separation involves *electrophoresis* and is based on the hypothesis that X- and Y-bearing sperm carry opposite electrical charges. If all the assumptions involved in this procedure are correct, when semen is placed in a chamber and direct current is run through it, the male-producing sperm will gather at one end of the electrode, female-producing sperm at the other. While it sounds as if some type of giant magnet were at work, the process is actually far more delicate than that. Sperm swim in whatever direction their heads are pointing, so the idea is to effectively "turn their heads." Again, researchers have had some limited success with animals, but results have been contradictory, and difficult to duplicate (theoretically because of slight differences in technique).

Still other methods are being investigated, most of them employing various types of filtration and sedi-

The Ericsson Method of Sperm Separation

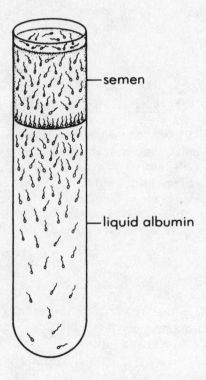

semen

liquid albumin

Source: Robert H. Glass and Ronald J. Ericsson, *Getting Pregnant in the 1980s* (Berkeley: University of California Press, 1982), p. 129.

mentation. Another that is currently of some interest involves immunization against one or the other sperm types. In one experiment, mouse sperm treated with anti-serum that would act against Y sperm succeeded in increasing the proportion of female births "slightly." Continuing research may very well prove more successful.

The "Girl" Methods

Until very recently there was little hope for increasing the female odds outside of timing within the menstrual cycle, but science marches on.

The most promising method was encountered by accident. Scientists discovered that when Dr. Ericsson's technique was used in the presence of the fertility drug *Clomid* (clomiphene citrate) the results were reversed; that is, an unusually high percentage of females were born. Investigators are still unsure why this is so, but they have also learned that other substances, such as the hormone gonadotrophin, will yield similar results.

In late 1983, two physicians, Stephen Corson and Frances Batzer, reported in *American Medical News* a new sperm separation technique for producing girls. Similar to Dr. Ericsson's process, this one ("devised by an Italian researcher") employs glycogen instead of albumin. At this point, too little data is available to assess its effectiveness, but perhaps it will eventually prove useful.

Selective Abortion

One of the most widespread, and certainly effective, methods of "sex control" among the ancients was the use of selective infanticide. In many parts of the world and at various points in history, newborns of the "wrong" sex (usually female) were promptly murdered or abandoned. In one Asian culture (the Ossetes of the Central Caucasus), for example, pregnant women were separated from their husbands until birth. If the new child was a girl, the mother simply returned to her husband empty-handed. During the Tokgawa period in Japan (1600–1868), some districts registered approximately nine male births for every one female, implying that seven or eight out of every nine females had been destroyed.

Of course we're far more civilized today. Very few parents would even dream of annihilating their newborn child because its sex was unsuitable, yet a fair number of them do not suffer such qualms *before* the child's actual birth. Now that a baby's sex can be determined well before delivery time, physicians are encountering abortion requests with increasing frequency.

Before continuing, I wish to point out that this is not a treatise on abortion in general. That issue is highly personal and much too complex to dismiss in a few brief paragraphs. In addition, even when one is addicted to either an ultraliberal or ultraconservative approach, moral attitude has been known to change abruptly in the face of personal confrontation. In other words, whatever you, or anyone, believes on a hypothetical level does not always apply to situations of blunt reality.

Selective abortion is quite another matter. While it is not my place to issue moral judgments (although I expect to be criticized for doing so), I cannot help but find this sort of value system too materialistic to digest. If a living room chair is the wrong shape or a new pair of shoes unsuitable, we return them to the store. But do we have the same "right" to, in essence, do the same with an unborn child? While there may be many more-or-less legitimate reasons for wishing to terminate an unwanted pregnancy, it is difficult to extend any such reasoning to a pregnancy of a specific sex.

The process of *amniocentesis* can be performed on a pregnant women by inserting a needle through the abdominal wall and withdrawing some of the amniotic fluid from the "bag of waters" that surrounds the fetus. The fluid is then examined for the presence of sex chromatin in addition to chromosomal disorders and other information. For a number of reasons this prenatal evaluation cannot be thought of as a routine procedure.

First, in spite of the fact that amniocentesis has been around for a number of years, it continues to carry some small, but very real, risk of death to the fetus or injury to the mother. (The incidence of spontaneous abortion as a result is less than one percent, however.) Second, the procedure can only be safely performed after sixteen weeks of pregnancy, and requires another two weeks to obtain all the results, putting fetal development well beyond the period when most physicians feel that abortion is relatively safe and simple.

Other methods of prenatal examination aren't much more satisfactory in this regard. *Ultrasound* offers the advantages of being cheaper, faster and safer than amniocentesis, but the earliest that fetal sex can be determined is after twenty-six weeks. Even after the fifth month, sex can only be ascertained in 90 percent of the patients.

Several years ago the Chinese developed a method of sex determination known as "Anshan aspiration." In this procedure, an aspirator is inserted into the pregnant woman's cervix to withdraw a little clump of sloughed-off cells, which are then examined microscopically. The evaluation can be performed as early as forty-seven days after conception and is reputed to be 93 percent accurate in forecasting fetal sex.

Essentially the same technique under the name of *chorionic villus biopsy* is now being tested in the United States and Europe, which could offer a number of advantages over amniocentesis in the event that abortion is indicated. The test is performed by suctioning out a small plug of tissue from the end of one or more villi, the hairlike branching material on the outside of the fetal sac, a procedure that *must* be performed between the eighth and tenth weeks of pregnancy since the villi begin to disappear after that time. The villus tissue is then analyzed for chromosomal and biochemical defects as well as sex, and results are available within a few days at the most. Examination at such an early point in pregnancy is a distinctly positive feature, but the method is still in the experimental stage at this time. However safe and reliable it turns out to be, it is unlikely that it would ever entirely replace amniocentesis because only the latter can reveal certain types of nerve defects.

As methods of prenatal sex determination continue to improve, the use of abortion as a means of sex selection presents an ever-growing concern. Surveys indicate that only about 5 percent of the physicians in this country are willing to perform abortions—or even amniocentesis—for this purpose. There is no way to accurately confirm that figure, however, since the answers of the remaining 95 percent are dependent on the doctors' basic honesty and disregard what percentage of them might be persuaded to deviate from their usual custom under particular circumstances. Further, there are already a number of cases on record where couples have requested amniocentesis, and even abortion, on the pretext of hereditary sex-linked disorders that did not in fact exist. Still more frightening is the possibility that couples may force a return to the days of "illegal abortions" with all their inherent potential dangers, and inevitably performed for exorbitant sums of money. (If the market is there, *someone* is going to reap a profit from it.)

It is perhaps because of this that Dr. M. Neil MacIntyre of Case Western Reserve University in Cleveland, one of the developers of amniocentesis, has performed his procedure for purposes of sex selection, even though he is personally opposed to it. Says Dr. MacIntyre: "A doctor's personal biases should not be imposed upon people by a genetic counselor like myself. If information is available, parents should be able to have it." Then, too, some physicians have proposed that there are benefits in learning ahead of time that they have produced the "wrong" sex because it gives them time to work through their disappointment before the baby is born.

But under other kinds of circumstances, the underlying concern is really the ethical implications of adopting such a casual approach to the termination of a developing human life. If parents can abort a pregnancy because its sex is unsuitable, should they have this same right if a detailed genetic analysis discloses the unborn child to be a dark-eyed brunette when they have in mind a blue-eyed blond? The ultimate prospects are overwhelming.

As the well-known pediatric psychologist, Dr. Lee

Salk, puts it: "It turns having a child into a shopping expedition. If you have such strong feelings about the sex of your child, you should think twice before taking on parenthood. Consider buying a poodle instead." In this instance, Dr. Salk is actually speaking of sex selection in general, but his remarks are particularly pertinent to the issue of selective abortion.

What If "The" Method Did Exist?

Many questions about human sex preselection remain to be answered, and two of them immediately come to mind here: If there were a foolproof or nearly foolproof method of choosing the sex of a child, would couples use it? If the method were accepted, what would be the impact on our society?

Many people naively assume that if we had an easily accessible means of controlling the sex of children all couples would use it. But judging by present attitudes and behavior change, this assumption is very much oversimplified.

First, sex predetermination techniques, assuming they require some advance planning and preparation, would work only for planned pregnancies, and current estimates are that approximately one half of all pregnancies occurring in this country are unplanned. Given that a large share of babies born each year in this country "just happen," we must acknowledge that even if all couples were theoretically in favor of sex predetermination, not all would use it. Second, a recent national study of some six thousand "ever married" women under age forty-five, conducted by Dr. Charles F. Westoff, professor of sociology and associate director of the Office of Population Research at Princeton

University, and Dr. Ronald Rindfuss, of the Center for Demography and Human Ecology at the University of Wisconsin, revealed that more women were *not* in favor of sex control than were supporting it. When asked the question, "Sometime soon, couples will be able to choose in advance whether they will have a boy or girl . . . How would you feel about being able to choose the sex of a child?" some 39 percent reacted favorably, 47 percent unfavorably, and the rest had no reaction.*

It is arguable that the percentage of "unfavorables" in such surveys might be even higher if the sex selection method involved artificial insemination (and in terms of the sperm separation studies done so far, only artificial insemination would be completely successful). In countries where machismo pressures affect the male ego, artificial insemination would probably not be a very popular route to parenthood. Artificial insemination could also raise questions in Catholic countries, because it requires masturbation to obtain the semen sample and might be considered an unnatural way to conceive.

Then, too, there is nothing very romantic about artificial insemination. It's a fairly safe assumption that younger couples and those who have been married only a short time would be less inclined to do their conceiving under laboratory conditions. Additionally, those who are ultimately anticipating a "typical" American family of two-children/one-of-each are generally aware that they stand a pretty good chance of achieving it by doing nothing at all (that is, nothing in

---

*This survey, and all others as far as I know, do not consider selective abortion as an acceptable means of sex selection. This "option" is therefore not treated as part of the data.

addition to engaging in their usual patterns of sexual intercourse).

For families that already include two or more children of the same sex and none of the other, it's a different story. Many couples who perhaps ten years earlier would not have been the least interested in sex selection are now changing their minds. Both Dr. Ericsson and Dr. Dmowski have noted that the overwhelming majority of their clients are already parents of two or three girls, who have come to them to "try for a boy."

Whether the converse will also occur after "girl methods" are more widely available is still unknown, of course, but we can venture a guess that it would be with somewhat less fervor. Statistically, the sex ratio of "last" children is 117:100 (compared, you will remember, to the overall birth rate of 105:100), indicating that more couples tend to "stop" after the birth of a son—whether he be an only, second, third, or tenth child.

It is difficult to judge the acceptance of an innovation before it is available (if a survey had been conducted before the automobile was invented, there would very likely have been a majority of horse-and-buggy supporters), but such speculation does tend to prevent us from assuming that everyone wants to preselect a baby's sex.

What Would the Impact Be?

Would sex control in any way contribute to the state of human health? Would the birth rate take a nose dive when people no longer had to have those "extra" children to balance out the sex ratio of their brood? Would we have an overwhelming excess of males? Is it possible that sex control could have some disastrous effects that would constantly remind us that "it's not nice to fool with Mother Nature?" Speculation ranges from the grimly serious to the almost ludicrous.

Realistically, we could expect a trend toward smaller families, at least in this country, thereby contributing significantly to current goals for population control. As I have already indicated, our national studies tell us that more couples with two children of the same sex plan to have a third than those with "one of each," and that those with only daughters are much more likely to seek a third child. When the first child is a boy, the interval between that birth and that of a second child is generally longer—usually some three months longer—than if a girl is the firstborn. In other words, parents of daughters are more eager to "try again."

In India, Korea, and other countries where an even greater premium is placed on male births, the introduction of sex control might have an even more significant impact on eliminating the "extra" children. Studies in Korea have shown that over 53 percent of women say they would continue having children until they had a son, and in Seoul an attitudinal study revealed that one-fourth of the women would allow their husbands to take a concubine if they themselves did not produce a son.

Such reports certainly suggest that sex control would lead to fewer births and more people "stopping at two," or even one. Nevertheless, human behavior being as erratic as it is, there is no guarantee that if couples could bear sons at will, they might not have *more* children. That consequence is more likely to occur in the less-developed nations of Asia, Africa, and

South America—where sons are viewed as income producers for the family—than in either the United States or Europe. But in any case, a significant excess of males in the population would eventually cause the birth rate to fall simply because there would be fewer individuals equipped with a uterus. Demographers have estimated that, all other things being equal, the birth rate would drop by 16 percent if the sex ratio shifted to 60:40 (men to women).

For better or worse, at this time all of the major surveys reveal a strong preference for males as either firstborn or only children regardless of the total number of children planned. Westoff and Rindfuss (who conducted the study on whether sex selection methods would be used at all) found a 63 percent preference for males. Another large study among college men and women showed an 85 percent preference. Because of a basic desire among Americans (and Europeans) for "balanced" families, we can assume that those with an even number of children—two, four, or even six—would probably contain half of each sex, if the parents had an opportunity to choose. But in odd-numbered families, the indications are that, for a while anyway, they would lean heavily toward boys: only children would more likely be boys; three-child families would tend to follow a pattern of boy-girl-boy, and so on.

Even taking into account that half of all pregnancies aren't specifically planned, and of the remaining half some portion would not use sex selection techniques, and that there will always continue to be, at best, some slight percentage of failures, the net impact would still result in a significant increase of males in the population—perhaps fifty-five to sixty males per forty or forty-five females. There is a chance the sex ratio could go even higher. And it is exactly that concern that has sociologists and so-called social activists wringing their hands.

Among their dire predictions about a heavily male population, and they haven't missed many, are the following: Prostitution, male homosexuality, and polyandry (multiple husbands) might become norms. There would be "raiding" of young women and girls by older men. Since males are reputed to be more aggressive, the crime rate would rise; there would be more wars, more alcoholism, lowered morality, decreased church attendance, and a reversion to "frontier-like" practices.

"All social life is affected by the proportion of the sexes," the demographer H. L. Greenberg has pointed out. "Wherever there would be a considerable predominance of one sex over the other, there would be less prospect of a well-ordered social life. Unbalanced numbers inexorably produce unbalanced behavior." The Columbia University sociologist Dr. Amitai Etzioni agrees. He points out that a preponderance of men could have profound social effects: since women read more and are generally more culturally oriented than men, a male-dominated society might see a decline in these activities and interests. Etzioni also notes that "men vote systematically and significantly more Democratic than women," so there might well be political changes. And there would surely be more sports on television.

There is a point at which it becomes difficult to take all of this seriously. However well-founded the fears may be, the line of thinking is simplistic for several reasons. First, it just isn't that likely that men are going to move back into caves simply because there are more of them than there are women. Second, by such time as a male majority might evolve, the women's movement will have become well enough established that they won't be idly standing by to watch the men "take over." Third, it ignores the probability that with fewer women available, the men will become more competitive for their attentions—striving to become better-educated, more successful, more culture-oriented, and so forth. And fourth, there is the simple law of supply and demand: a shortage of any commodity raises its value. It is reasonable—indeed, probable—to expect that any temporary "shortage" of women will be followed by a temporary "boom." Eventually, after vascillating for a time, the ratio can be expected to settle into a fairly even balance.

In the meantime, we could probably cope. In Alaska, where there is a ratio of 132:100 (males to females), there appears to be no excess of either criminal behavior or homosexuality compared to other states. Further, it's too soon to tell yet what kind of effect the women's movement will have on such existing factors as alcoholism, for example. Traditionally, the disease has been higher among males; in recent years the rate has been rising among females. We cannot accurately predict, therefore, that an increase in the future adult male population would necessarily result in an increase in alcoholism.

For the elderly, there is a definite bright spot in the predicted "boy boom." At the present time the male:female ratio is about equal among people of "reproductive" age. By age 65 there are only 72 males for every 100 females. As life expectancies continue to lengthen, there would doubtless be a good many older women delighted to see an "excess" of males.

A very real concern is the likelihood of a dramatic shift in birth order, with child number one being almost exclusively male. It's possible that such a system could deal a severe blow to the drive for female equality, not to mention the psychological impact on all those girls as they learned they were only "second choice." Fueling the fire of sex-role stereotypes is the significant fact that firstborn children are most likely to be intelligent and successful, while their younger brothers and sisters tend to be more sociable and dependent, ambitious and highly motivated.

Studies consistently find that firstborn and only children have predominated in American colleges at least as far back as 1874, particularly in the "prestige" schools. Firstborn and only children are found in disproportionate numbers among high scorers on the National Merit Scholarship test, on the list of distinguished American scientists, and in *Who's Who in America*. The most common explanation for this finding is that first and only children receive more of their parents' time and attention than subsequent children do. They begin to interact with adults sooner, gain verbal ability sooner.

Whether or not a listing in *Who's Who* is a sign of "success" in life is a matter of opinion, but there is much evidence to suggest that firstborn children have the edge on achievement in general. As things stand right now, girls have an equal chance at the firstborn role. With the availability of sex determination techniques, this situation would certainly change, at least temporarily. But noted anthropologist Margaret Mead had another point to add: those daughters who are born will at least have been *chosen*, not merely serving as stepping stones en route to the ultimate goal of a son.

An added concern is that some parents who carefully and scientifically map out their plans for "one girl baby" and "one boy baby" will greet their newborn children with a whole group of expectations set in cement. The boy is to be their achiever; he is going to go out and conquer the business world and make his mommy and daddy mighty proud. The girl is going to be their princess; she will be lovely, feminine, marry a wonderful man, provide grandchildren, and generally be the perfect complement to their ambitious son. Needless to say, this would not do very much to enhance our recent progress in the shedding of traditional sex roles.

Finally, even a system of "perfect" sex selection will have some flaws, some room for human error. At the moment the game of sex selection roulette is still chancy enough so that most couples are psychologically prepared for either a boy or a girl, no matter how seriously they plan. Lack of such preparation could lead to family misery when an "error" does occur.

And another possible psychological problem to think about: What would happen if husband and wife could not agree on the sex of their children? Would what previously was a matter of fate be the subject of a furious fight? (You may recall that this was the case with Mimi and Brian, mentioned in Chapter 1.) Would these matters have to be settled, perhaps legally in contract form, prior to a marriage ceremony?

Once we consider some of these ramifications, we can see why not everyone is enthusiastic about the possibility of sex predetermination. Although no religious organization or other group has ever condemned research in this area, it is certainly the fear of consequences that has inhibited efforts along these lines. Dr. Hans Zeisel, professor of law and sociology at the

University of Chicago, has expressed his concern: "I have always thought that this is the type of discovery that should not be made. The mere possibility of destroying this natural balance carefully developed over millions of evolutionary years is dangerous. . . . One need not be a religious person to be in awe of such natural constants, and to fear the wrath of the gods if they are tampered with." The journal *Science* has sounded a similar note of caution: "The obvious problems that are likely to arise as a result of such experiments make one wonder whether human beings have yet acquired wisdom to make use of such powers." Some people have gone so far as to suggest that governments should suppress research in this area, much in the way they might urge an end to research for ever more powerful bombs which could someday blow up in our faces.

But there is another side to that issue, too. Writing in the *American Journal of Medical Genetics,* Laurence E. Karp reminds us that "there is more to fear from a society that would suppress individualism to the point of forbidding sex preselection than from a society that could tolerate such a practice."

Not everyone is pessimistic. There is the distinct probability that after a temporary surge of male births and firstborn male children, females would again "come into style" and eventually the normal overall balance would be reachieved, the only difference being that individual couples would retain the ability to choose their own children's sex.

We cannot ignore the positive effect on health, given that sex-linked diseases such as hemophilia and Duchenne muscular dystrophy could be all but eliminated. These diseases and others are "carried" by the female but affect only male children. A woman who knew she was a carrier could use sex selection techniques to ensure that she had only daughters.

Smaller families would help relieve couples of some of the less-rewarding aspects of parenthood, perhaps sparing fathers some of the financial pressure they often endure, affording greater opportunities because there are fewer children, and allowing mothers more freedom to pursue their other needs and interests.

Whatever the implications—demographic, social, personal—of a near-perfect method of sex preselection, one thing is clear. We are talking about a new dimension on man's control over life, one that undoubtedly offers some benefits but that carries with it the burden of responsible decision-making. In the early 1970s, when there was increasing acceptance of the philosophy that not everyone has the potential to be a good parent, and that all of us should think seriously about whether or not to have a child instead of assuming that parenthood follows marriage as the night the day, many couples became conscious of that burden of decision for the first time. Adding the option of sex selection will make that burden heavier.

We must hope that as medical technology evolves further in this direction, mankind will evolve too, toward emotional maturity and an increased concern about the effects of our behavior on the lives of others.

Appendix

Questions and Answers

I've heard that having only boys or only girls "runs in families," and that some of us are preprogrammed to have one sex or the other. Is that true?

There is no reason to believe that the probability of having a son or the probability of having a daughter is influenced by your family background. Remember, when you are dealing with fifty-fifty odds, the laws of probability dictate that certain families will be all boys or all girls. For instance, if we select random families of five children, one in every thirty-two of them will consist of all sons or all daughters. If you randomly choose families with ten children, every 1,024 will have either all boys or all girls.

A friend of mine claims that she could predict that her first and third pregnancies were boys because of the way she carried the baby. Is there a difference in the position of the male and female fetus in the uterus?

You're bound to hear old wives' tales of this nature, but the fact is that fetal position and the way the baby is "carried" do not reflect the sex of the unborn child.

My cycles are between thirty and thirty-two days long. Is there anything abnormal about this, and will the fact that my cycles are long affect my chances of having a boy baby?

There is a significant variation in the female menstrual cycle, with the typical twenty-eight-day cycle representing only the average. You have no reason for concern because your cycles are somewhat longer than the average. In a thirty-two-day cycle, ovulation would occur around day 18 and your "boy days" five or so days before that. You'll want to keep careful track of your basal body temperature readings for more precise timing.

I am trying to pinpoint the "girl day" of my cycle, and take my temperature almost every morning. Once in a while I oversleep—or simply forget to take it. How should I record the forgotten day on my chart?

Just leave that day blank. Missing a temperature reading for one or two days a month—as long as those missed days are not around the time of ovulation, when you are looking for a sudden dip and rise in temperature—probably won't confuse your overall chart. If you find you often forget about taking your temperature until it's "too late," try taping a little note on the face of your alarm clock, so it's the first thing you see when you wake up.

Is it true that using "the Pill" can increase your chances of never having children?

No, at least not that we know of for the overwhelming majority of women who use it. On the other hand, when you've been using the oral contraceptive for a few years, and then suddenly stop, your body can be temporarily confused. It may take you two or three months to get back "on schedule."

Are there any do-it-yourself chemical tests to detect when ovulation is about to occur?

A few years ago "test tapes" for determining changes in the cervical mucus became popular. But they're not recommended today, primarily because they're not reliable. Your best bet in predicting ovulation is to follow your basal body temperature graph and note the changes in the discharges of cervical mucus through your vagina.

How often does twinning occur?

About one out of every eighty births involves twins, and about one-third of these are identical twins. The older a woman is and the more children she has had, the higher the probability that she will have twins. In addition, fraternal twinning is affected by heredity. If your mother or grandmother had fraternal twins, you are more likely to have them than a woman whose family has no such history (twinning does not "skip generations," as is often said). No hereditary influence is operative in the birth of identical twins.

How does twinning occur?

If for some reason your ovary works overtime during a cycle and releases more than one egg during ovulation, it is possible that two or more eggs will be fertilized. When this dual type of sperm-egg union occurs, the resulting babies may not look alike at all—one may be a boy and the other a girl. This is fraternal twinning, in which each of the babies grows from its own fertilized egg.

When only one egg is fertilized and soon afterward splits into two separate parts, each part containing exactly the same type of materials, the result is identical twins. These look-alike children have exactly the same chromosome makeup and share equally in the contributions of their mother and father.

How can I plan for a healthy pregnancy?

Ideally you should find a physician before you become pregnant. Ask if there is any particular medication either of you should avoid while you're seeking a pregnancy. There is evidence, for instance, that certain drugs interfere with spermatogenesis or can have an adverse effect if taken early in pregnancy. It's best to check on them.

What about immunization for German measles?

Of utmost importance during your preconception physical exam is a rubella (German measles) evaluation. Rubella is a common, mild infectious disease of childhood. For many years it was assumed to be an atypical form of measles or scarlet fever. But in the early 1940s it was discovered that exposure to rubella during the first three months of pregnancy can have a disastrous effect on the developing child (the other two diseases, though they can be extremely serious, do not have this effect). Cell division is somehow inhibited, and the child may be born with such congenital defects as deafness, cardiac malformation and/or cataracts. Be sure you are immune to rubella! The chances are over 80 percent that you already are. You were most likely exposed to the disease when you were a child. It's highly infectious yet also very mild, so you may not have known you had it. Ask for a rubella screening test. It may take a couple of weeks to get the results, so plan accordingly. Don't try to conceive or allow conception to occur until you get the results. If you do *not* have rubella antibodies in your system, or if there is some doubt, you should get the vaccination as soon as possible *and* postpone conception for at least three months after the immunization (which actually gives you a mild case of the disease).

Should I give up smoking during my pregnancy?

Yes! Smoking should be avoided during pregnancy— during the entire length of the pregnancy. Both epidemiological and experimental studies unanimously support the view that smoking has a retarding effect on fetal growth. Analyses of hundreds of thousands of births have shown that the average birth weight of babies born to smoking mothers is a full 6.1 ounces less than that of babies born to mothers who didn't smoke during their pregnancies. Also, significantly more babies under five pounds are born to women who smoke.

The problems associated with low birth weight are well documented. These babies are often disadvantaged from the moment of birth through the early years of their lives, and maybe longer. A large study conducted in England concluded that "the mortality in babies of smokers was significantly higher than that of non-smokers." The same study raised questions about the long-term effect of smoking during pregnancy on those babies who survive: children of smokers followed up during their early years were found to be significantly shorter and to have low ratings of "social adjustment" and greater frequency of reading retardation. It's not smart to smoke any time, but during pregnancy it's really unforgivable.

And it is not just the mother-to-be who should kick the habit before conception is even considered. The prospective father should, too. The effect of exhaled cigarette smoke on a fetus has not yet been fully measured, but there is reason to believe that it could also be harmful. Besides, after the child is born, you'll be very conscious of the adverse effect exhaled smoke can have on growing children, particularly with regard to the development of respiratory problems.

Does painful menstruation mean painful pregnancy?

For the most part, the conditions that produce pain in menstruation have nothing to do with pain in pregnancy or difficulty in childbirth. In most cases no connection between the two is to be expected. For most women pregnancy is not painful, although there may be some discomfort.

I've heard that large doses of vitamin E increase male potency and fertility and may help you have a son. Is that so?

Not so. If you're eating a well-balanced diet, you have absolutely no need for vitamin E supplements.

There is no relationship between vitamin E intake and male fertility, potency, or the probability of having a son. The rumor that there is such a connection stems from some laboratory animal experiments in which vitamin E was eliminated from the diet. These animals did develop fertility problems (they also developed scaly tails, but no one has yet made a human analogy here). But there is no evidence that just because a lack of some nutrient causes a problem, an excess of it will offer extra benefits.

Does drinking coffee prior to intercourse improve a man's chances of fertilizing an egg with a male-producing sperm?

Certainly not. If you enjoy a cup or two of coffee before bedtime—and it doesn't keep you up all night—then by all means have it. But do not expect that you can "stimulate" either type of sperm into action with coffee or any other food or drink.

If I want a boy baby, should I eat lots of "alkaline" foods?

No, this rumor is simply a new addition to the growing lore of food faddism. Eat a well-balanced diet and forget the nonsense about acid and alkaline foods.

How long can you postpone parenthood and still have a successful, healthy pregnancy?

Maybe you've heard some of the old wives' tales (or, more appropriately, old mothers' tales) that make a woman at age 29.9 feel as if she's over the hill. But before you panic, consider the facts. Generally speaking, first pregnancies in the early thirties and subsequent pregnancies in the late thirties present no greater risks than those that occur when the mother is in her twenties. In the majority of cases the timing of parent-hood is a socially rather than a medically oriented decision.

There are some caveats here. A woman's fertility may decline as she gets older. One thing is obvious. If you wait until you are thirty-five or so to seek a first pregnancy, you are going to have less time to work out a fertility problem if one does come up. Additionally, there is an increased incidence of mongolism among births to women over thirty.

What is mongolism and how often does it occur?

Children affected by mongolism are usually phys-ically and mentally deformed and have a reduced life span. There is a definite association between maternal age and risk of mongolism. A woman under age thirty runs about a 1-in-1,500 risk of having a mongoloid child; the chances are 1 in 750 births at ages thirty to thirty-four, and 1 in 280 births at ages thirty-five to thirty-nine. The risk goes up to 1 in 130 (or, according to some sources, a 1-in-100 chance) between forty and forty-four. This correlation between advancing mater-nal age and mongolism applies to both first and subse-quent births.

Is any major religious group opposed to techniques of sex predetermination?

Not that I'm aware of. On the other hand, many individuals have serious ethical or philosophical doubts about man's interfering with nature's ways.

Are there any medical side effects associated with following your advice on increasing the odds on a male or on a female birth?

No, with the exception that, as I pointed out, in seeking a boy baby you'll be focusing sexual intercourse on a relatively unfertile portion of the menstrual cycle. This will mean that it may take a few more months to conceive. Planning for a girl baby is easier, since the "girl days" coincide with the time of maximal fertility.

Are we close to the time when there will be a diaphragm or condom that is able to screen out X or Y sperm?

No, that idea is just theoretical at this point.

Is it true that taking hot baths or wearing tight undershorts can both decrease male fertility and reduce the chances of having a son?

In cases of marginal fertility, when the man has a relatively low sperm count, it is possible that tight underwear (which would press the testes close to the body, and thus raise the temperature of these sperm-producing glands) or repeated exposure to hot water could further reduce fertility. But there is no reason to believe that male-producing sperm would be more affected than female-producing ones.

Is there any particular position in sexual intercourse that favors the conception of a boy baby or of a girl baby?

No. Some earlier reports suggested that there were advantages to altering coital positions to favor a child of a specific sex, but I know of no evidence to suggest that this is true.

If normal body temperature is 98.6, why is the basal body temperature so much lower, and why does it go up so sharply after ovulation?

Your body temperature drops below 98.6 when you are in a deep sleep. That's why it's relatively low immediately upon awakening. It is the presence of increased amounts of progesterone in your bloodstream after ovulation that makes your temperature go up.

Glossary

ACIDIC	A sour or sharp substance. Opposite of alkaline.
ALKALINE	Having a salt base. Opposite of acid.
AMENORRHEA	The failure to menstruate. May be either primary (failure in ovarian function) or secondary (due to another cause, such as stress, endocrine imbalance, or surgical removal of the uterus).
AMNIOCENTESIS	A procedure in which a small amount of the amniotic fluid surrounding the fetus is removed for analysis prior to

birth. Mongolism and a number of other genetic syndromes can be identified in this manner. Similarly, the sex of an unborn child can be detected, although the procedure is not routinely used for that purpose.

AMPULLA
The dilated, central portion of the Fallopian tube which curves around the ovary and is connected to the infundibulum; the storage place (or "sperm reservoir") for sperm prior to ejaculation.

ANDROGEN
Any substance that stimulated male characteristics. Testosterone is an androgen.

ANSHAN ASPIRATION
A method of prenatal testing, developed by the Chinese, in which cells suctioned from the uterus can be examined for genetic disorders as well as fetal sex. The procedure is similar to chorionic villi biopsy.

ANTENATAL SEX DETERMINATION
Prediction of the sex of the unborn child after conception but before birth.

ARTIFICIAL INSEMINATION
The introduction of semen into a woman's vagina or cervical canal by artificial means.

BARTHOLIN'S GLANDS
The glands located within the vagina which produce mucus secretions to keep the vagina moist.

BASAL BODY TEMPERATURE	The body temperature reading which is obtained by using a thermometer every morning upon awakening before engaging in any type of physical activity.
BULBOURETHRAL GLANDS	See COWPER'S GLANDS.
CASTRATION	The removal of the male testes or the female ovaries.
CELL	The fundamental, microscopic unit of living substance which alone or with other cells performs the body's basic functions.
CERVIX	The narrow opening at the neck of the uterus.
CHORIONIC VILLI BIOPSY	A still experimental method of prenatal testing for chromosomal and biochemical disorders, in addition to fetal sex. A small plug of tissue is removed from the end of one or more chorionic villi, the hairlike projections of the membrane that surrounds the embryo during early pregnancy, which is then examined microscopically.
CHROMOSOMES	The material contained in the nucleus of the cell, composed essentially of DNA (deoxyribonucleic acid). DNA determines the heredity-related

characteristics of the child.

CILIA

Tiny hairlike projections capable of lashing movement; those, for instance, found on the lining of the inside walls of the Fallopian tubes.

CLEAVAGE

The cell division immediately following fertilization.

CLIMACTERIC

Events including menopause which result in the termination of reproductive functioning.

CLITORIS

The pea-shaped organ in the female located just above the urethra. The clitoris has many sensitive nerve tissues becauses it plays a major part in female orgasm. It is often considered the female counterpart of the male penis.

CONCEPTION

The merging of the female egg sex cell (ovum) and the male sex cell (sperm) in the Fallopian tube.

CORPUS LUTEUM

Also known as the "yellow body." The name for the ovarian follicle when it takes on a new function after ovulation. The corpus luteum produces both progesterone and estrogen.

COWPER'S GLANDS

Male glands that secrete mucus fluids along the urethra during sexual excitement.

CYTOPLASM

The cell exclusive of the nucleus.

DEMOGRAPHER

A person involved in the statistical study of population topics such as births, deaths, migration, and marriage patterns.

DOUCHE
The rinsing out of the vagina with a syringe or similar device. Not a form of birth control.

DOWN'S SYNDROME
See MONGOLISM

DUCTUS DEFERENS
See VAS DEFERENS.

ECTOPIC PREGNANCY
A serious medical condition in which a fertilized egg becomes implanted in the Fallopian tube or somewhere else other than the uterus.

EMBRYO
The developing baby during its first two months, after which it is called a fetus.

ENDOCRINE
The adjective applied to organs that secrete substances into the blood or lymph systems to produce a specific effect on another organ or part.

ENDOMETRIOSIS
A condition in which portions of the lining of the uterus travel to and attach to other parts of the pelvic region. A common cause of female sterility.

ENDOMETRIUM
The tissue-and-blood inner lining of the uterus which goes through cyclical changes to prepare for the possibility of implantation. When implantation occurs, the endometrium provides nourishment and protection for the growing baby.

EPIDEMIOLOGY
The science that focuses on the

occurrence, distribution, and types of disease in a population.

EPIDIDYMIS
The long-celled tubes near the testes where the sperm mature.

ESTROGEN
A basic female hormone produced by the follicle in the ovary, responsible for the development of the female's secondary sex characteristics and for the growth and maintenance of the uterus, Fallopian tubes, and vagina.

ESTRUS CYCLE
Heat cycles of most nonhuman animals which ensure that intercourse and ovulation occur at or about the same time.

FALLOPIAN TUBES
The two tubes with fingerlike fringes which attract the egg when it has been released from the ovary and serve to transport it to the uterus.

FETAL DEATH
The expulsion of a fetus which shows no sign of life. A stillbirth. Generally statistically reported only after the twentieth week of pregnancy.

FETUS
The name given to the growing baby from the end of the second month of pregnancy until birth.

FIMBRIA
The fingerlike fringes of the Fallopian tubes which serve to attract the egg into the tubes once ovulation has occurred.

FOLLICLE (OVARIAN)
The structure in the ovary in which the egg cells grow.

FRATERNAL TWINS	Twins resulting from the simultaneous fertilization of two eggs; fraternal twins need not be of the same sex, and they have different genetic makeups.
FSH	Follicle stimulating hormone, released by the pituitary gland. In the female it acts directly on the ovary, causing an egg within the follicle to begin to grow; in the male it acts on the testes to stimulate spermatogenesis.
GENE	Determinant for a hereditary trait.
GLAND	An organ that produces a specific product or secretion.
GONAD	A specific sex gland such as an ovary or a testis.
GONADOTROPIC	The adjective that describes those hormones which serve to stimulate either the ovary or the testis.
HORMONE	A substance produced by a special type of gland to control functions of other organs.
HUMAN CHORIONIC GONADOTROPIC HORMONE (HCG)	A hormone secreted by the placenta. Serves to maintain functioning of the corpus luteum. HCG's presence in the urine is a common sign of pregnancy.
HYALURONIDASE	An enzyme released by sperm to chemically break down the protective layer of the egg (the zona pellucida).

HYPOPHYSIS	See PITUITARY GLAND.
IDENTICAL TWINS	Twins that develop from the same egg; identical twins are always of the same sex and have the same genetic makeup.
IMPLANTATION	The embedding of a fertilized egg in the tissues of the lining of the uterus, the endometrium.
IMPOTENCE	The inability of the man to participate in sexual intercourse.
INGUINAL CANAL	The canal in the groin through which the testes descend into the scrotum prior to birth.
INSEMINATION	The introduction of male sex cells into the woman's body, through either sexual intercourse or artificial means.
INTERSTITIAL CELL-STIMULATING HORMONE (ICSH)	The master gland hormone in the male which stimulates the production of testosterone by the testes; identical chemically to luteinizing hormone (LH) in the female.
INTROITUS	The entrance to the vagina.
LABIA MAJORA	Two rounded folds of tissue which extend from the mons pubis downward throughout the area of the vulva.
LABIA MINORA	The small lips. Two parallel folds of soft tissue which begin at the clitoris and end in the lower vulva area.
LUTEINIZING HORMONE	A hormone produced by the pituitary gland to stimulate the

release of an egg from the follicle. LH also plays a role in the
development and functioning of
the corpus luteum, or yellow
body. LH is identical chemically to the male hormone
ICSH.

MEIOSIS Cell division which reduces the
number of chromosomes in the
nucleus of the cell to half their
original number.

MENSTRUATION The shedding of the lining of the
uterus (endometrium) when
pregnancy has not occurred.

MITTELSCHMERZ A cramplike pain in the abdomen experienced by some
women at or near the time of
ovulation.

MONGOLISM A genetic disease that leaves a
child both mentally and phys-
ically deformed, with a reduced
life span.

MUCORRHEA The disintegration of the
mucus-cervical plug resulting in
a whitish discharge from the vagina.

NIDDAH A practice of Orthodox Jews
whereby sexual intercourse is
avoided for seven full days following the termination of the
menstrual flow.

OOCYTE A cell which will differentiate
into a mature ovum.

OVARY The egg- and hormone-producing sex glands (gonads) of the female.

OVIDUCTS
See FALLOPIAN TUBES.

OVULATION
The process whereby the egg is released from the ovary.

OVUM
The egg cell produced about every month between puberty and menopause by the female sex gland, the ovary.

pH
The commonly used measure of alkalinity and acidity. The neutral point is pH 7. Above pH 7 alkalinity increases; below pH 7 acidity increases.

PITUITARY GLAND
Also known as the hypophysis, or master gland. A small gland in the base of the brain which secretes hormones that regulate many human systems.

PRIMARY SEX RATIO
The number of male conceptions per one hundred female conceptions

PROGESTERONE
The hormone of pregnancy, produced by the ovary's follicle after ovulation. Acts together with estrogen to coordinate and regulate the events of the menstrual cycle.

PROLIFERATIVE PHASE
That portion of the menstrual cycle which follows the menstrual flow and precedes ovulation. The proliferative phase is characterized by increased levels of estrogen.

PROSTAGLANDIN — A substance within the male semen which appears to increase the muscular activity of the uterus.

PROSTATE GLAND — A gland in the male near the bladder and the urethra which secretes a special type of fluid that aids in the maintenance and movement of sperm.

RUGAE — The small folds of skin in the vaginal canal which stretch and enlarge during childbirth.

SCROTUM — The fleshy pouch which contains the male testes and related organs.

SECONDARY SEX RATIO — The number of male births per one hundred female births.

SECRETORY PHASE — That portion of the menstrual cycle which follows ovulation and ends with the first day of the menstrual flow. The secretory phase is characterized by increased secretion of progesterone until midphase.

SEMINAL VESICLES — The two small sacs located near the base of a man's bladder which secrete a special type of fluid that gives the sperm added mobility.

SEX RATIO — See PRIMARY SEX RATIO and SECONDARY SEX RATIO.

SPERMATOCYTE — A cell which will differentiate into a mature sperm call.

SPINNBARKEIT — From the German, meaning

"ability to be drawn out into a thread"; used to describe the quality of the cervical mucus just prior to ovulation.

STEROID — Adjective used to describe the common chemical structure of sex hormones.

TESTOSTERONE — A male sex hormone produced by the testes which, among other things, controls maturation in the male and the functioning of his reproductive system.

THERMAL SHIFT — The rise in basal body temperature (by a degree or more) in the day or days just after ovulation.

ULTRASOUND — A method of prenatal testing based on the principle that sound vibrations are reflected at varying frequencies according to the density of the tissue at which they are directed. The reflections create an image, called a sonogram, that is useful in detecting structural abnormalities before birth, as well as aiding in the process of amniocentesis.

URETHRA — The tube which carries urine from the bladder to the outside of the body; in the male, the urethra also serves to conduct sperm.

UTERUS — Also known as the womb. The

hollow pear-shaped organ in the center of the female abdomen where a growing baby receives protection and nourishment.

VAGINA   The muscular tube which serves as both the female organ for sexual intercourse and the birth canal.

VAS DEFERENS   The duct that carries sperm from the testes to the ejaculatory duct.

ZONA PELLUCIDA   The outer membrane of the female egg cell which serves in a protective capacity.

ZYGOTE   The name given to the new cell formed by the joining of an egg and sperm.

Selected References

FOR HISTORICAL PURPOSES ONLY

Benedict, A., *Why We Are Men and Women*. New York: Ross and Company, 1929.

Buzzacott, F., *Mystery of the Sexes: Secrets of Past and Future Human Creationism*. Chicago: Advanced Thought Publishing, 1914.

Calhoun, L. A., *The Law of Sex Determination and Its Practical Application*. New York: Eugenics Publishing Company, 1910.

Carr, E., *Choosing the Sex of Children*. New York: Theo Carr Publishers, 1938.

Conway, J. W., *The Science of Sex Control*. Kansas: Norton Champion Press, 1919.

Cox, C. S., *The Cause and Control of Sex*. Los Angeles: The Austin Publishing Company, 1923.

235

Daniell, J., "Sex-Selection Procedures," *Journal of Reproductive Medicine* 28:4, April 1983.

Dawson, E. R., *The Causation of Sex in Man*. London: H. K. Lewis, 1909 (and 1917).

Dechmann, L., *Within the Bud*. Seattle: Washington Printing Company, 1916.

Erskine, J. M., *Sex at Choice*. London: Christophers, 1925.

Gordon, A.D.G., "Bicarbonate for a Boy, Vinegar for a Girl," *Nursing Times*, May 4, 1978.

Hoffman, H. W., *Sterility and Choice of Sex in the Human Family*. Privately printed, 1916.

Kraft, F., *Sex of Offspring. A Modern Discovery of a Primeval Law*. Cleveland, Ohio: Barsuette Company, 1908.

Langendoen, S., and W. Proctor, *The Pre-Conception Gender Diet*. New York: M. Evans and Company, Inc., 1982.

Lorrain, J., "Pre-conceptional Sex Selection," *Int. J. Gynaecol. Obstet*. 13:127–130, 1975.

Mathison, R. R., *The Eternal Search*. New York: G. P. Putnam's Sons, 1958.

MacFadden, B., and C. Clinton, *Practical Birth Control and Sex Predetermination*. New York: MacFadden Book Company, 1935.

McConnel, Mrs. D., *Race Making: A Practical Natural Method of Self Determination and Control*. London: Health for All, 1920.

McElrath, P. J., *The Key to Sex Control*. New York: privately printed, 1911.

Okland, F., *Is It a Boy: Sex Determination According to Superstition and Science*. London: George Allen & Unwin, 1932.

Ostrander, S., and L. Schroeder, *Natural Birth Control and How to Choose the Sex of Your Child*. (Originally published as *Astrological Birth Control*.) New York: Bantam Books, 1973.

Reed, T. E., *Sex: Its Origin and Determination*. New York: Rebman Company, 1913.

Rorvik, D. (with Landrum B. Shettles), *Your Baby's Sex: Now You Can Choose*. New York: Dodd, Mead, 1970.

————, *Choose Your Baby's Sex*. New York: Dodd, Mead, 1977.

Sandell, D. H., *Boy or Girl: How Parents Can Decide the Sex of Their Child*. New York: Fortuny's Publishers, 1938.

Schenk, L., *The Determination of Sex*. Chicago: Werner Company, 1898.

Starkweather, G. B., *Law of Sex*. London: J. & A. Churchill, 1883.

Stolkowski, J., and J. Lorrain, "Preconceptial Selection of Fetal Sex," *Int. J. Gynaecol, Obstet,* 18:440–443, 1980.

Stolkowski, J., and J. Choukroun, "Preconception Selection of Sex in Man," *Israel Journal of Medical Sciences* 17:1061, 1981.

Sylvan, F., *Natural Painless Childbirth and the Art of Determination of Sex*. New York: Dutton, 1916.

Taber, C. W., *Suggestion: The Secret of Sex*. Chicago: Charles Kerr and Co., 1899.

Terry, S. H., *Controling Sex in Generation*. New York: Fowler and Wells, 1885.

Tucker, W., *Do You Wish to Choose the Sex of Your Children?* London: Bale Company, 1925.

von Borosini, A., *Choosing the Sex of Your Child*. New York: Exposition Press, 1953.

Wang, C. T., *Human Sex Control*. Taiwan: Taipei Books, 1960.

RESEARCH DOCUMENTS

Asdell, S. A., "Time of Conception and Ovulation in Relation to the Menstrual Cycle," *Journal of the American Medical Association,* August 13, 1927.

Barlow, P., and C. G. Vosa, "The Y Chromosome in Human Spermatozoa," *Nature* 226:961, 1970 (June).

Beernink, F., and R. J. Ericsson, "Male Sex Preselection Through Sperm Isolation," *Fertility and Sterility* 38:4, October 1982.

Benendo, F., "The Problem of Sex Determination in the Light of Personal Observations," *Polish Endocrinology* 21:200, 1970.

Bertstein, M. D., "Parental Age and the Sex Ratio," *Science (N.Y.)* 118:448, 1953

————, "Studies in the Human Sex Ratio," *Journal of Heredity* 45:59, 1954.

————, "Semen Separation Technique Monitored with Greater Accuracy by B-body Test," *Int. J. Fertility* 24:4, 1979.

Bhattacharya, B. C., *et al,* "Successful Separation of X and Y Spermatozoa in Human and Bull Semen," *Int. J. Fertility* 22:30–35, 1977.

Billings, E. L., *et al,* "Symptoms and Hormonal Changes Accompanying Ovulation," *Lancet,* February 5, 1972, p. 282.

Birnholz, J. C., "Determination of Fetal Sex," *New England Journal of Medicine* 309:16, October 20, 1983.

Blackman, A. *The New York Times,* September 6, 1978, p. 10.

Bochkov, N. P., and A. A. Kostrova, "Sex Ratio Among Human Embryos and Newborns in a Russian Population," *Humangenetik* 17:91, 1973.

Boczkowski, L., "Abnormal Sex Determination and Differentiation in Man," *Obstetrics and Gynecology* 41:310, 1973 (February).

Boutelle, Ann, "Suspense in Pregnancy," *Vogue,* Vol. 68, September 1978.

"Boys or Girls?" *AMA Brief Reports* (pub. by the Journal of the American Medical Association), November 18, 1983.

Brody, J., "Political Imbalance Is Foreseen If Sex of Offspring Is Controlled," *The New York Times,* September 15, 1968, p. 57.

————, "Survey Finds Boys Preferred as the First-Born, Girls as the Second," *The New York Times,* May 4, 1974.

Brower, K-H., *et al,* "The Frequency of Y Chromatin-Positive Spermatozoa During *in Vitro* Penetration Tests under Various Experimental Conditions," *Fertility and Sterility* 28:10, October 1977.

Campbell, C., "The Manchild Pill," *Psychology Today,* Vol. 10, August 1976.

Caughley, G., "Offspring Sex Ratio and Age of Parents," *Journal of Reproductive Fertility* 25:145, 1971.

Cederqvist, L. L., and F. Fuchs, "Antenatal Sex Determination," *Clinical Obstetrics and Gynecology* 13:159, 1970.

"Choosing the Baby's Sex," *British Medical Journal,* February 2, 1980.

Ciocco, A., "Variations in the Sex Ratio at Birth in the United States," *Human Biology* 10:36, 1938.

Clare, J., and C. Kiser, "Social and Psychological Factors Affecting Fertility: Preferences for Children of a Given Sex," *Milbank Memorial Quarterly* 29:621, 1952.

Cohen, M., "Differentiation of Sex as Determined by Ovulation Timing," *International Journal of Fertility* 12:32, 1967.

Cohen, M., *et al,* "Spinnbarkeit: A Characteristic of Cervical Mucus," *Fertility and Sterility* 3:201, 1952.

Cook, R., "Sex Control Again in the News," *Journal of Heredity* 31:270, 1940.

Cruz-Coke, R., "Birth Control and Sex Ratio," *Lancet* 2:426, 1970 (August 22).

Dahlberg, G., "Do Parents Want Boys or Girls?" *Acta Genetica Statistica Medica* 1:163, 1948.

Decker, A., and W. H. Decker, *Passport to Parenthood* (booklet). Privately printed, 1971.

Delepine, J., "*Good Housekeeping* Gave Us Our Son," *Good Housekeeping,* Vol. 195, August 1982.

Diasio, R. B., and R. H. Glass, "Effects of pH on the Migration of X and Y Sperm," *Fertility and Sterility* 22:303, 1971.

Dinitz, S., *et al,* "Preference for Male or Female Children: Traditional or Affectional?" *Marriage and Family Living* 15:128, 1964 (May).

Dmowski, W., *et al,* "Use of Albumin Gradients for X and Y Sperm Separation and Clinical Experience with Male Sex Preselection," *Fertility and Sterility* 31:1, January 1979.

"Do Cool Incubators Make Male Sea Turtles?" *Science News,* Vol. 116, December 8, 1979.

Dove, G. A., and C. Blow, "Boy or Girl—Parental Choice?" *British Medical Journal,* December 1, 1979.

Elstein, M., *et al,* editors, *Cervical Mucus in Human Reproduction.* Copenhagen: Scripton, 1973.

Ericsson, R. J., *et al,* "Isolation of Fractions Rich in Human Y Sperm," *Nature* 246:421, 1973.

Etzioni, A, "Sex Control, Science and Society," *Science* 161:1107, 1968.

Evans, J. M., *et al,* "An Attempt to Separate Fractions Rich in Human Y Sperm," *Nature* 253:352, 1975.

Ewert, R. J., "Sex Ratio and Sex Determination," *British Medical Journal* ii:358, 1918.

"Female Baby Choice Now Possible," *American Medical News,* October 28, 1983.

Fletcher, J. C., "Ethics and Amniocentesis for Fetal Sex Identification," *New England Journal of Medicine* 301:10, September 6, 1979.

Fox, C., *et al,* "Continuous Measurement by Radio-Telemetry of Vaginal pH During Human Coitus," *Journal of Reproduction and Fertility* 33:69, 1973.

Fox, C. A., and B. Fox, "A Comparative Study of Coital Physiology with Special Reference to the Sexual Climax," *Journal of Reproductive Fertility* 24:319, 1971.

Frazer, J., *The Golden Bough.* New York: Macmillan, 1935.

Freedman, D., *et al,* "Size of Family and Preferences for Children of Each Sex," *American Journal of Sociology* 116:141, 1960.

Fuchs, F., "Genetic Amniocentesis," *Scientific American* 242:6, June 1980.

Galton, L., "Decisions, Decisions, Decisions," *New York Times Magazine,* June 30, 1974.

Gebre-Medhin, M., *et al,* "Association of Maternal Age and Parity with Birth Weight, Sex Ratio, Stillbirths and Multiple Births," *Environmental Child Health,* Vol. 22, 1976.

Glass, R., "Sex Preselection," *Obstetrics and Gynecology* 49:1, January, 1977.

Glass, R. H., and R. J. Ericsson, *Getting Pregnant in the 1980s.* Berkeley: University of California Press, 1982.

Goodwin, J. M., "Season and Sex Ratio," *Lancet* 1:652, 1971 (March 27).

Gordon, M., "The Control of Sex," *Scientific American* 199:87, 1958.

Gray, E., and D. K. Morgan, "Desired Family Size and Sex of Children," *Journal of Heredity* 67:319, 1976.

Guerrero, R., "Time of Insemination in the Menstrual Cycle and Its Effects on the Sex Ratio Thesis," Harvard School of Public Health, Boston, 1968.

————, "Sex Ratio: A Statistical Association with Type and Time of Insemination in the Menstrual Cycle," *International Journal of Fertility* 15:221, 1970.

————, "Association of the Type and Time of Insemination Within the Menstrual Cycle with Human Sex Ratio at Birth," *New England Journal of Medicine* 291:(20)1056, 1974 (November 14).

————, "Type and Time of Insemination Within the Menstrual Cycle and the Human Sex Ratio," *Studies in Family Planning* 6:367, 1975.

Guerrero, R., and C. A. Lanctot, "Aging of Fertilizing Gametes and Spontaneous Abortion," *American Journal of Obstetrics and Gynecology* 107:263, 1970.

Gunby, P., "Sex Selection Before Child's Conception," *Journal of the American Medical Association* 241:12, March 23, 1979.

Guttmacher, A., *Life in the Making.* New York: Viking Press, 1933.

Hamilton, W. D., "Extraordinary Sex Ratios," *Science* 156:477, 1967.

Harlap, S., "Gender of Infants Conceived on Different Days of the Menstrual Cycle," *New England Journal of Medicine* 300:26 June 28, 1979.

Harrison, G. A., *The Structure of Human Populations.* Oxford: Clarendon Press, 1972.

Hartman, C., *Science and the Safe Period.* Baltimore: Williams and Wilkins, 1962.

Heath, C. W., "Physique, Temperament and Sex Ratio," *Human Biology* 26:336, 1954.

Helitzer, F., "Do You Want a Boy or Girl?" *Princeton Alumni Weekly,* May 21, 1974.

Hobbins, J. C., "Determination of Fetal Sex in Early Pregnancy," *New England Journal of Medicine* 309:16, October 20, 1983.

Hooper, J., "Making Girl Babies," *Omni,* September 1983.

Howkins, J., and G. Bourne, *Shaw's Textbook of Gynaecology.* London: Churchill-Livingston, 1971.

"The Implications of Sex Preselection," Human Reproduction, *Technology Review,* Vol. 82, March/April 1980.

Irwin, T., "Boy or Girl: Would You Choose Your Baby's Sex?" *Parents' Magazine,* November 1970, p. 67.

Jablon, S., and H. Kato, "Sex Ratio in Offspring of Survivors Exposed Prenatally to the Atomic Bomb in Hiroshima and Nagasaki," *American Journal of Epidemiology* 93:253, 1971.

James, W. H., "Cycle Day of Insemination, Coital Rate and Sex Ratio," *Lancet,* January 16, 1971, p. 112.

———, "Coital Rate, Sex Ratio and Season of Birth," *Lancet,* July 17, 1971, p. 159.

———, "Gonadotrophin and Sex Ratio," *Lancet,* 1980.

———, "Sex Ratio in Negroes," *Annals of Human Biology* 2:4, 1975.

———, "Sex Ratio and the Pill," *Lancet,* May 12, 1973.

———, "Sex Ratios in Large Sibships in the Presence of Twins and in Jewish Sibships," *Journal of Biosocial Science* 7:165, 1975.

———, "Timing of Fertilization and Sex Ratio of Offspring—A Review," *Annals of Human Biology* 3:6, 1976.

Kahn, H., and A. Weiner, "Towards the Year 2000: Work in Progress," *Daedalus,* Summer 1967.

Karp, L. E., "The Arguable Propriety of Preconceptual Sex Determination," *American Journal of Medical Genetics* 6:185, 1980.

Keseru, T. L., *et al,* "Oral Contraception and Sex Ratio at Birth," *Lancet,* March 2, 1974.

Keyfitz, N., "How Birth Control Affects Births," *Social Biology* 18:109, 1971.

Kleegman, S. J., "Therapeutic Donor Insemination," *Fertility and Sterility* 5:7, 1954.

————, "Can Sex Be Predetermined by the Physician?" *Excerpta Medica* 199:109, 1966.

Kolata, G., "First Trimester Prenatal Diagnosis," *Science,* Vol. 221, September 9, 1983.

Lake, A., "Selecting the Sex of Babies: The New Moral Dilemma," *McCall's* 103:47, July 1976.

Largey, G., "Sex Control and Society: A Critical Assessment of Sociological Speculations," *Social Problems* 20:310, 1973.

Lieberman, E. J., "A Doctor Forecasts Determining of Sex of Child in Advance," *The New York Times,* November 27, 1968, p. 27.

Lyster, W. R., "Three Patterns of Seasonality in American Births," *American Journal of Obstetrics and Gynecology* 110:1025, 1971.

Lyster, W. R., and M. H. Bishop, "An Association Between Rainfall and Sex Ratio in Man," *Journal of Reproductive Fertility* 10:35, 1965.

MacMahon, B., and T. Pugh, "Sex Ratio of White Births in the United States During the Second World War," *American Journal of Human Genetics* 6:284, 1954.

McCartney, E., "Sex Determination and Sex Control in Antiquity," *American Journal of Philology* 43:62, 1922.

Markle, Gerald, "Sex Ratio at Birth: Values, Variance and Some Determinants," unpublished manuscript, 1973.

Markle, G. E., and C. B. Nam, "The Impact of Sex Predetermination on Fertility," *Population Index* 36:319, 1970. Summary of paper presented at the 1970 meetings of the Population Association of America.

————, "Sex Predetermination: Its Impact on Fertility," *Social Biology* 18:73, 1971 (March).

Martin, L., "Your Child's Sex—Can You Choose?" *Parents*, Vol. 56, October 1981.

Martin, W. J., "Sex Ratio During War," *Lancet* 2:807, 1943.

Mason, A., and N. G. Bennett, "Sex Selection with Biased Technologies and Its Effect on the Population Sex Ratio," *Demography* 14:3, August 1977.

Mawe, E. S., "Type of Nuchal Hair and a Possible Theory of Prediction of Sex," *Journal of Anatomy*, July, 1911.

"May Change Girl to Boy, Says Huxley," *New York Herald*, January 20, 1922.

Mikamo, L., "Prenatal Sex Ratio in Man," *Obstetrics and Gynecology* 34:710, 1967.

Mittwoch, U., "Do Genes Determine Sex?" *Nature* 221:446, 1969.

Moghissi, K., "Cyclic Changes of Cervical Mucus in Normal and Progestin-Treated Women," *Fertility and Sterility* 17:663, 1966.

"More Boy Babies in Post-War Years," *Statistical Bulletin*, Metropolitan Life Insurance Company 20:1, 1939.

"More Childless Wives Conceive Through Use of Frozen Sperm," *The New York Times*, January 8, 1979.

Mortimer, D., and D. W. Richardson, "Sex Ratio of Births Resulting from Artificial Insemination," *British Journal of Obstetrics and Gynaecology* 89: 132, February 1982.

Muehleis, M. S., and S. Y. Long, "The Effects of Altering the pH of Seminal Fluid on the Sex Ratio of Rabbit Offspring," *Fertility and Sterility* 27:12, December 1976.

Newcomb, S., *The Probability of Causes of the Production of Sex in Human Offspring*. Washington: Carnegie Institute, 1904.

Odell, W. D., and D. L. Moyer, *Physiology of Reproduction*. St. Louis: The C. V. Mosby Company, 1971.

Pakrasi, K., and A. Halder, "Sex Ratio and Sex Sequences of Births in India," *Journal of Biosocial Science* 3:377, 1971.

Parkes, A., "Mythology of the Human Sex Ratio," in *Sex Ratio at Birth—Prospects for Control.* American Society of Animal Science, 1971 (symposium held at the Pennsylvania State University, University Park, Pennsylvania).

Pearl, R., and R. N. Salaman, "The Relative Time of Fertilization of the Ovum and the Sex Ratio Among Jews," *American Anthropologist* 15:668, 1913.

"Periodic Abstinence: Sex Preselection—Not Yet Practical," The George Washington University Medical Center *Population Reports,* Series 1, No. 2, May 1975.

Pohlman, E., "Statistical Evidence of Rationalization: Preferences for Sex of Child," *Psychological Reports* 20:1180, 1967.

————, "Some Effects of Being Able to Control Sex of Offspring," *Eugenics Quarterly* 14:(4)274, 1967 (December).

Prospects for Sexing Mammalian Sperm, ed. by R. P. Amann and G. E. Seidel, Jr. Boulder: Colorado Associated University Press, 1982. (Report of international conference held in Denver on March 19–20, 1982.)

Quinlivan, W. L. G., *et al,* "Separation of Human X and Y Spermatozoa by Albumin Gradients and Sephadex Chromatography," *Fertility and Sterility* 37:1, January 1982.

Revelle, R., "On Rhythm and Sex Ratio," *New England Journal of Medicine* 29:1083, 1974.

Rohde, W., *et al,* "Gravitational Patterns of the Y-Bearing Human Spermatozoa in Density Gradient Centrifugation," *Journal of Reproduction and Fertility* 42:587, 1975.

Rose, K., "Can You Pre-select the Sex of Your Child?" *Harper's Bazaar,* Vol. 108, July 1975.

Rosenfield, A., *The Second Genesis: The Coming Control of Life.* Englewood Cliffs, N.J.: Prentice-Hall, 1969.

Rostron, J., and W. H. James, "Maternal Age, Parity, Social Class and Sex Ratio," *Ann. Human Genetics* 41:205, 1977.

Rothschild, "X and Y Sperm," *Nature* 187:253, 1960.

Rubin, E., "The Sex Ratio at Birth," *American Statistician* 21:45, 1967.

Russell, W. T., "Statistical Study of the Sex Ratio at Birth," *Journal of Hygiene* 36:25, 1936.

Sampson, J. H., *et al*, "Gender after Induction of Ovulation and Artificial Insemination," *J. Androl.* 4:43, 1983.

Schellen, A., *Artificial Insemination in the Human*. Amsterdam: Elsevier Company, 1957.

Schnall, M., "Electronmicroscopic Study of Human Sperm," *Fertility and Sterility* 3:62, 1952.

Schuster, D., and L. Schuster, "Study of Stress and the Sex Ratio," Proceedings, 77th Annual Convention, American Psychological Association, Vol. 4, 1969, p. 335.

"Selecting the Sex of Your Infant," *Science News,* Vol. 115, March, 3, 1979.

"Sex Determination," *Science* 126:1059, 1957.

Shearer, M., *et al,* "The Sex Ratio of Offspring Born to State Hospitalized Schizophrenic Women," *Journal of Psychiatric Research* 5:349, 1967.

Sheps, M., "Effects of Family Size and Sex Ratio on Preferences Regarding the Sex of Children," *Population Studies* 17:66, 1963.

Shettles, L. B., "X and Y Spermatozoa," *Nature* 187:254, 1960.

Shino, P. H., *et al,* "Sex of Offspring of Women Using Oral Contraceptives, Rhythm, and Other Methods of Birth Control Around the Time of Conception," *Fertility and Sterility* 37:3, March 1982.

Simpson, J. L., "More Than We Ever Wanted to Know About Sex—Should We Be Afraid to Ask?" *New England Journal of Medicine* 300:26, June 28, 1979.

Snyder, R. G., "The Sex Ratio of Offspring of High Performance Aircraft Pilots," *Human Biology* 33:1, 1961.

Stephens, J. D., and S. Sherman, "Determination of Fetal Sex by Ultrasound," *New England Journal of Medicine* 309:16, October 20, 1983.

Sullivan, W., "Sperm Screening in Lab May Help Produce Boys," *The New York Times,* December 28, 1973, p. 1.

Tarver, J. D., and C. Lee, "Sex Ratio of Registered Live Births in the United States," *Demography* 5:347, 1968.

Taylor, M., "Sex Ratio of Newborns: Associated with Prepartum and Postpartum Schizophrenia," *Science* 164: 723–724, 1969.

Taylor, M., and R. Levine, "The Interactive Effects of Maternal Schizophrenia and Offspring Sex," *Biological Psychiatry* 2:274, 1970.

Teitelbaum, M. S., "Factors Associated with the Sex Ratio in Human Populations," in Harrison, G. A., *The Structure of Human Populations.* Oxford: Clarendon Press, 1972.

Teitelbaum, M., and N. Mantel, "Socio-Economic Factors and the Sex Ratio at Birth," *Journal of Biosocial Science* 3:23, 1971.

"Testing Fetuses," *Time,* Vol. 115, March 24, 1980.

Uddenberg, N., *et al,* "Preference for Sex of the Child Among Pregnant Woman," *Journal of Biosocial Science* 3:267, 1971.

Vilinskas, J., "Clinical Studies in Sex Pre-Determination," *The Woman Physician* 26:419, 1971.

"War and Sex Ratio," *Statistical Bulletin,* Metropolitan Life Insurance Company 30:5, 1949.

Weatherbee, C., "Toward Preselected Sex," *Science News* 94:118, 1968.

Westoff, C. F., and R. R. Rindfuss, "Sex Pre-Selection in the United States: Some Implications," *Science* 184:633, 1974.

Whelan, E., "Can You Control Your Baby's Sex?" *Modern Bride,* June/July 1974.

———, *A Baby? . . . Maybe: A Guide to Making the Most Fateful Decision of Your Life.* New York: The Bobbs-Merrill Company, 1975.

———, "Human Sex Ratio as a Function of Insemination Timing Within the Menstrual Cycle," *Social Biology,* December, 1975.

Winston, S., "The Influences of Social Factors upon the Sex Ratio at Birth," *American Journal of Sociology* 37:1, 1931.

———, "Birth Control and the Sex Ratio at Birth," *American Journal of Sociology* 38:225, 1933.

Wittels, I., and P. Bornstein, "A Note on Stress and Sex Determination," *Journal of Genetic Psychology* 124:333, 1974.

"Women: The Next Endangered Species?" *Mademoiselle,* Vol. 101, May 1983.

Index

249